Statistical Design
and Analysis
of Clinical Trials
Principles and Methods

Chapman & Hall/CRC Biostatistics Series

Published Titles

Chapman & Hall/CRC Biostatistics Series

Statistical Design and Analysis of Clinical Trials
Principles and Methods

Weichung Joe Shih

Rutgers University
Piscataway, New Jersey, USA

Joseph Aisner

Rutgers Cancer Institute of New Jersey
New Brunswick, New Jersey, USA

CRC Press
Taylor & Francis Group
Boca Raton London New York

CRC Press is an imprint of the
Taylor & Francis Group, an **informa** business

A CHAPMAN & HALL BOOK

CRC Press
Taylor & Francis Group
6000 Broken Sound Parkway NW, Suite 300
Boca Raton, FL 33487-2742

ISBN 13: 978-1-4822-5049-7 (hbk)

Visit the Taylor & Francis Web site at
http://www.taylorandfrancis.com

and the CRC Press Web site at
http://www.crcpress.com

Contents

Preface

Clinical trials, as an enterprise, reflect the work of many participants and the expertise they bring to bear: biologists, toxicologists, pharmacologists, medical investigators, research nurses, project managers, computer programmers, database specialists, medical writers, health authority regulators, and, of course, biostatisticians. One need only attend an annual conference of the Society for Clinical Trials to discover a network of participants from many different disciplinary areas who all contribute to clinical trials. This book, however, concentrates on the biostatistics component of the enterprise.

Most of this book is based on the teaching material that we used for public health and medical students, residents, and fellows over the past 15 years. In addition to our academic experience, we also worked on clinical trials sponsored by pharmaceutical companies and governmental health organizations. We benefited from the experience of working with teams on a wide variety of clinical development projects, and we found that the biostatistics component of clinical trials is truly an integration of many fundamental scientific principles and statistical methods. Chapter 1 is an overview, which begins with ethical and safety principles, criteria for quality studies, and classification of different types of clinical trials. Chapters 2 and 3 cover core trial design concepts. Many design issues in clinical trials stem from the fact that a clinical trial needs to balance the two aspects of its nature: scientific experiment and clinical practice. For a scientific experiment, validity (Chapter 2) and efficiency (Chapter 3) are the main considerations. Students using this book need some basic knowledge in hypothesis testing and confidence intervals to learn, in Chapter 4, the principles and methods of sample size and power calculation. Thus, the fundamental principles of probability and inferential statistics are prerequisites for using this book. Regarding analytical methods, students must learn regression, analysis of variance and covariance, analysis of categorical data, longitudinal data, and survival data. However, a one-semester course in clinical trials is neither just an overview of statistical methods, nor can it cover these methods in depth. We cover the fundamental analysis of covariance and stratified analysis in Chapter 5 and leave many other topics of methods in the appendices of other related chapters. Almost all modern clinical trials involve data monitoring and interim analyses. We devoted Chapters 6 through 8 to sequential designs and methods, from two-stage Phase II cancer trials to Phase III group sequential trials, including monitoring safety, futility, and efficacy. Following the sequential trials and interim analyses, a more recent topic is the monitoring and modification of the maximum information in the middle of a clinical trial. In Chapter 9, we discuss the development of sample size reestimation and adaptive group sequential procedures, but only briefly, because this subject remains an open research area. We end the book with a discussion of missing data in Chapter 10. Missing data is not totally avoidable, but it should and can be minimized by proper trial design and responsible trial conduct. Missing data is an old issue, but a recent report from the National Research Council has brought the importance of this issue again into the spotlight. In Chapter 10, we discuss some matured methods and one newly developed method under different assumptions regarding the nature of the missing data. The sequence of the chapters is based on our view of a logical progression of concepts and technical levels as taught in our courses. We move from design concepts, sample size calculation, to analytical methods including ANCOVA, then to trial monitoring with sequential designs, interim analyses, adaptive midcourse modification, and finally we give special attention to the ubiquitous problem of missing data. Some instructors may rearrange the sequence or supplement with other topics according to individual preference. In all chapters, in-class discussions and exercises are held for the students to practice. Many examples are from trials published in medical journals or our consulting projects. Where computation is required, we provide instructions for acquiring and using an online software program; we also introduce simple commands using R functions or SAS® procedures for some techniques, although some homework assignments also train students to carry out computer simulations.

Our training and work experience in both academia and industry, as well as in consulting to governmental health authorities, allow us to present teaching material that reflects different aspects of clinical trials that may be oriented to academic research, commercial development, or public health. However, finding the proper level and coverage was a challenge. Because this course was taught in a public health and medical school environment, it is interesting to observe that some concepts such as control of confounding and bias were relatively easy to grasp for students from epidemiology, whereas the essence and calculation of critical values and study power were relatively comprehensible for students from the biostatistics program. Hence, to provide a balanced set of homework assignments, in-class exercises, and examinations for the whole class was a concern for us. In addition to having different disciplinary backgrounds, students were often at different stages of their academic or career pursuits. For example, in the same class, we saw students who were about to finish their master's degrees and were searching for a job in the pharmaceutical or biotech industry, mixed with students who had already acquired a Master of Science or a Master of Public Health degree and were in the second or third year of their doctoral programs. In some semesters, the course also attracted pharmacy students or physicians in their residency or fellowship programs from the medical school or the university cancer center. They certainly extended the classroom discussions to another dimension, especially for review and critique of the medical literature, which we often excerpted as part of the teaching material.

Input from students and colleagues allowed us to develop and focus the course material. The result, we believe, spans the spectrum of those who deal with clinical trials directly and those who read and interpret the material. For the student of statistics, we believe this work places in context the specific principles and methods applicable to clinical trials, and the mathematical exercises illustrate the process. For the clinicians who engaged in the course, we further believe that, even if the formulae and their derivation seemed daunting, the course helped to focus their understanding of how clinical data are collected, monitored, and analyzed. Importantly, the study of bio-statistics of clinical trials helps us develop vital collaborators to the team of investigators. In addition, the study of biostatistics helps the clinical investigator understand what the statistical methods can provide. Educated consumers of biostatistics make better investigators and furthermore develop their critical reading skills. To that end, statistical critiques are now often included in the Oncology Fellows' Journal Club presentations at the Rutgers Cancer Institute of New Jersey.

Because this book is based on our teaching material over the years, our primary goal for the book is to serve as a text for colleagues teaching clinical trials in a similar academic setting. As a text for a one-semester course, there are certainly materials that we chose to omit in this first edition, such as sub-group analysis and multiple tests and comparisons. Thus, we leave plenty of opportunity in this book for other colleagues to fill in and improve upon.

To students, we hope that you find this book an enjoyable read and that you learn from it. To fellow teachers, we hope that you find this book a useful text for your class.

Acknowledgments

We sincerely thank the many students and colleagues who participated in our teaching and our working experience in clinical trials. We are grateful for the opportunity developed in the setting of the Rutgers University School of Public Health and the Rutgers Cancer Institute of New Jersey, which provided the setting, support, colleagues, and students from whom we learned so much. In particular, we would like to thank our colleagues Irving K. Hwang, Gordon K. K. Lan, Dirk F. Moore, Yong Lin, Yujun Wu, and Pamela Ohman-Strickland, who have lectured with us at one time or another. We would also like to acknowledge Tina Chang Young, a student of this course (Spring 2013) and now a Doctor of Public Health candidate at the Rutgers School of Public Health, who read the initial and final drafts and provided numerous suggestions that improved the clarity of this book.

Weichung Joe Shih
Department of Biostatistics
Rutgers School of Public Health & Rutgers Cancer Institute of New Jersey
Rutgers, The State University of New Jersey

Joseph Aisner
Medical Oncology
Robert Wood Johnson Medical School & Rutgers Cancer Institute of New Jersey
Rutgers, The State University of New Jersey

Authors

Weichung Joe Shih, PhD, is professor and chair of the Department of Biostatistics, Rutgers School of Public Health, Rutgers University, New Brunswick, New Jersey, and director of Biometrics Division at the Rutgers Cancer Institute of New Jersey, New Brunswick, New Jersey. He is an elected fellow of the American Statistical Association and an elected member of the International Statistical Institute. Prior to joining academia, he spent his formative years at Merck Research Laboratories, Boston, Massachusetts. He served in the Advisory Board of the US FDA for reviewing new drug applications, and was associate editor of professional journals, including *Statistics in Medicine, Controlled Clinical Trials, Clinical Cancer Research, Statistics in Biopharmaceutical Research*, and *Statistics in Bioscience*. He has collaborated extensively with physicians in various therapeutic areas and authored numerous papers in statistical methodology in clinical trials. His research interests include adaptive designs and missing data issues.

Joseph Aisner, MD, is a professor of medicine and a professor of environmental and occupational medicine at the Robert Wood Johnson Medical School of Rutgers University, New Brunswick, New Jersey, director of Medical Oncology Unit at the Robert Wood Johnson University Hospital, New Brunswick, New Jersey, and co-leader of the Clinical Investigations Program at the Rutgers Cancer Institute of New Jersey. He has published extensively and has served on the editorial board of multiple journals, including *Journal of Clinical Oncology, Cancer Therapeutics, Medical Oncology, Clinical Cancer Research*, and *Hematology-Oncology Today*. He is a fellow of the American College of Physicians and the American Society of Clinical Oncology. He serves on and chairs several National Data Monitoring Committees, has served on multiple National Institutes of Health (NIH) Study Sections, and has headed two National Cooperative Cancer Study Groups. His research interests include cancer clinical trials and evaluation of therapeutic interventions.

1

Overview

Before we start, consider these two questions:

- Who was the pioneering British clinician who established the link between smoking and lung cancer?
- Who was the principal investigator who first used a randomized controlled clinical trial to test streptomycin in the treatment of pulmonary tuberculosis in 1940?

1.1 What Is a Clinical Trial?

In this book, we define *clinical trial* as "an experiment that studies the relationship between a disease or condition and a medical intervention for prevention, diagnosis, or treatment using human subjects." The ultimate goal of a clinical trial should be to advance medical knowledge and to improve medical practice to benefit the patients.

To better appreciate this definition, we will first answer the two questions posed above: The correct answer to both is *Sir Austin Bradford Hill* (1897–1991), Dean of the London School of Hygiene and Tropical Medicine (1955–1957). Hill conducted two types of clinical studies, both involving human subjects; however, the first study, linking smoking and lung cancer (1950), was based on observational investigations and the second, prospectively testing streptomycin in the treatment of pulmonary tuberculosis, was an experiment, that is, a clinical trial.

Clinical studies conducted in medical schools include retrospective surveys of clinical data or accumulated case reports, which are often cross sectional, as well as *clinical trials*, which are always prospective and thus require both a baseline and a follow-up period. Not all clinical studies are clinical trials, but all clinical trials are also clinical studies.

In Hill's article on statistical methods "General Summary and Conclusions" (1937), he states that "in both clinical and preventive medicine, and in much laboratory work, we cannot escape from the conclusion that ... many of the problems we wish to solve are statistical and that there is no way of dealing with them except by the statistical method." This statement highlights the critical role of statistics in the medical sciences. In other words, biostatistical methods have become one of the fundamental tools in the evaluation of medical information.

Many, but not all, statistical principles and methods used in clinical trials are also applicable to other types of clinical studies. A statistician or an epidemiologist should distinguish the nature of the study, in order to properly interpret the result. The statistical analysis is thus the tool for understanding results and meanings in all forms of clinical studies. Statisticians, epidemiologists, and even clinical trialists need to understand the statistical tools that they rely on for interpreting the data, much like a carpenter needs to understand what a hammer can or cannot do.

Some authors have defined a clinical trial as "a prospective study comparing the effect and value of interventions against a control in human beings" (Friedman, Furberg, and DeMets 1996). In our opinion, this describes a requirement for a *good* clinical trial, but it is a restrictive definition that excludes a large portion of clinical trials that are conducted without *concurrent controls*. We certainly are interested in good clinical trials. In fact, to understand what constitutes a good clinical trial is a central objective of this book. Certainly many investigators would object if we said that a single-arm dose-finding study in cancer patients was not a clinical trial. As an example of a clinical study that led to medical knowledge and defined the standard of care in a noncontrolled setting, consider the Papanicolaou test for cervical cancer, which reduced the disease-specific mortality from cervical cancer by nearly 70% from early 1930 to 1974 (Cramer 1974, Michael 1999). The path to medical knowledge is a process in which different levels of evidence are developed by different types of clinical studies, as summarized in Table 1.1. Randomized, controlled trials are certainly at the highest level in the hierarchy of evidence.

1.2 Requirements for a Good Experiment

An experiment should always be conducted by the primary investigator under and initial set of well-defined conditions and procedures. For a clinical trial, this set of conditions and procedures should be documented in a protocol. The trial protocol also serves as the operational manual for all participating investigators and staff to follow. This system is akin to an operational method in any laboratory experiment.

1.2.1 Discussion

Read the following excerpt from the Book of Daniel 1:1–16 (606 BC), which may be the earliest mention of a clinical study with dietary intervention in ancient history.

TABLE 1.1

Hierarchy of Evidence for Intervention Studies

Type of Evidence	Level of Evidence	Description
Systematic review of randomized, controlled trials or meta-analysis	1 (highest)	A synthesis of evidence from all relevant randomized, controlled trials (RCTs) with homogeneity
Individual randomized, controlled trial	2	An experiment in which subjects are randomly assigned to a treatment group or control group
Individual cohort study or a clinical trial without randomization or without control group	3	Cohort study: a follow-up observational study of a group(s)/cohort(s) to determine the development of an outcome(s) such as a disease, or an experiment in which subjects are not randomly assigned to a treatment group or control group
Case-control	4	Case-control study: a retrospective comparison of subjects with a condition or event (case) with those who do not have the condition or event (control) to determine characteristics (such as a treatment exposure) that might predict or alter the condition
Systematic review of qualitative or descriptive studies of series of cases	5	A synthesis of evidence from qualitative or descriptive studies to answer a clinical question
Expert opinion without explicit critical appraisal or consensus	6 (lowest)	Authoritative opinion of expert committee

Source: Burns PB, et al. *Plastic and Reconstructive Surgery* 128: 305–310, 2011; Melnyk BM and Fineout-Overholt E, *Evidence-Based Practice in Nursing and Healthcare: A Guide to Best Practice*. Lippincott, Williams & Wilkins, 2010.

In the third year of the reign of Jehoiakim king of Judah, Nebuchadnezzar king of Babylon came to Jerusalem and besieged it.... Then the king (of Babylon) ordered Ashpenaz, chief of his court officials, to bring into the king's service some of the Israelites from the royal family and the nobility—young men without any physical defect, handsome, showing aptitude for every kind of learning, well informed, quick to understand, and qualified to serve in the king's palace. He was to teach them the language and literature of the Babylonians. The king assigned them a daily amount of food and wine from the king's table. They were to be trained for three years, and after that they were to enter the king's service.

Among those who were chosen were some from Judah: Daniel, Hananiah, Mishael and Azariah.

But Daniel resolved not to defile himself with the royal food and wine, and he asked the chief official for permission not to defile himself this way. Now God had caused the official to show favor and compassion to Daniel, but the official told Daniel, "I am afraid of my lord the king, who has assigned your food and drink. Why should he see you looking worse than the other young men your age? The king would then have my head because of you."

Daniel then said to the guard whom the chief official had appointed over Daniel, Hananiah, Mishael and Azariah, "Please test your servants for ten days: Give us nothing but vegetables to eat and water to drink. Then compare our appearance with that of the young men who eat the royal food, and treat your servants in accordance with what you see." So he agreed to this and tested them for ten days.

At the end of the ten days they looked healthier and better nourished than any of the young men who ate the royal food. So the guard took away their choice food and the wine they were to drink and gave them vegetables instead.

In-Class Discussion: Could this story be viewed as a clinical study—and as a clinical trial? What information can you provide to support your answer? In your opinion, was it a "good" clinical trial? Why or why not?

1.2.2 Essential Steps of a Clinical Trial

More details will be discussed in later chapters, but the following outlines the essential steps of a clinical trial:

- Idea inception: The idea of a trial comes from a scientific rationale and a medical need to address. Investigators also have to catch the window of opportunity for conducting a clinical trial: public awareness of the disease burden, which is related to generating adequate interest for the study. If untested procedures are already accepted as the standard practice, it may be too late to propose a clinical trial. In proposing a clinical trial, some funding agencies may require the investigator to submit a short *letter of intent* (LOI), which is a brief outline of the essential elements of a trial protocol including rationale, objectives, participants, methods, and initial estimates of sample size and study duration. (See Homework 1.1 for sample LOI excerpts.)

- Planning: Planning includes preparing the study protocol, calculating the sample size, arranging study sites, and contracting personnel. It also includes having appropriate regulatory paperwork approved, such as the Investigational New Drug (IND) Application by the Food and Drug Administration (FDA), obtaining local institutional review board (IRB) review and approval, ensuring medical supplies and equipment, budgeting, case report form (CRF) preparation, and assessment of feasibility in subject numbers and other resources for initiating and conducting the trial.

- Conduct and monitoring: This step includes screening, enrolling, scheduling, and administering study intervention to subjects. It also involves data collection, completing the CRFs, and database management. Monitoring ongoing clinical trials is necessary because trials are very expensive in monetary costs and human resources, and thus careful monitoring is critical to ensure the trial's quality and ethics.

- Data analysis: Data analysis actually starts at the study planning stage when sample size and statistical methodologies are prepared, as well as during the ongoing trial monitoring. Upon completion of the trial, statistical analyses will yield study results for interpretation.

- Report writing and publication: There is a popular saying that "a job is never finished until all the paperwork is done." For industry-sponsored trials, a clinical study report (CSR) is written by the trial sponsor and submitted to health agencies for commercial license approval. Journal publications help to inform the medical community of the results; these publications also often serve as a marketing vehicle for manufacturers. For trials sponsored by research grants from government organizations and foundations such as the National Institutes of Health (NIH), Department of Veterans Affairs, Department of Defense, and National Science Foundation, the study report and journal publication are documentation for grant accounting. In other words, these publications serve as the "deliverables" of the grant.

- Next phase trial: Trials sponsored by industry often involve a series of steps in the New Drug Application (NDA) strategy. A trial's outcome likely affects other related trials in the NDA package. Completed academic trials can often result in new or revised hypotheses. In either case, scientific knowledge is advanced by clinical trials. The ultimate goal of all clinical trials should thus be to advance medical knowledge and to improve medical practice to benefit the patients.

Statisticians need to participate in each of these steps. The statistician in a clinical trial needs to be more than a consultant. In fact, he or she should be a full-fledged member of the investigative team and must take responsibility for the scientific integrity of the study, as well as make assessments of its safety, efficacy, and futility. As Ederer (1979) noted, a statistician engaged in a clinical trial should be prepared to become both a student of the science and a teacher for the use of statistics during the course of the study. This process entails studying and learning in detail the clinical subject matter and, often, teaching fundamental statistical and research concepts to collaborators.

1.2.3 Essential Sections of a Clinical Trial Protocol

The protocol for the trial is the central document that guides the study throughout the course of the work and serves as the roadmap. It is also an operations manual and must therefore be written in excruciating detail, especially for multicenter trials, in order to ensure consistency across sites where any ambiguity may lead to differences in interpretation. A complete protocol usually contains the following sections (details of some topics are discussed in later sections or chapters):

- Introduction: Includes rationale and purpose of the trial (i.e., background and significance).
- Objectives and endpoints: Includes scientific hypotheses (primary and secondary) to test and specific aims to accomplish.
- Design: Includes randomization, blinding, control treatment, sample size, and study duration.
- Patient eligibility: Inclusion and exclusion criteria, used to define the subject population. These criteria will impact, in part, the future generalizability of the trial results.
- Conduct procedures and visit schedule: Dose and dose adjustment, lab and clinical examination schedule, patient withdrawal guidance, and trial flowcharts for more complex trials.
- Measurements: Assessment criteria for clinical and laboratory findings to measure the outcomes in efficacy and safety.
- Statistical considerations: Includes sample size justification, randomization process (if pertinent), study monitoring and interim analysis (if applicable), and methodology for statistical analyses and handling of missing data.
- Quality control and assurance procedures.
- Appendices: Include informed consent form, references or medical criteria/definition of response, quality of life or other questionnaires if applicable, and so on.

1.2.4 Definition of a Well-Designed Study and Guidance for Evaluating a Protocol

Baumgardner (1997) summarized the fundamental requirements for a well-designed clinical trial as follows:

- Clear, definable, and relevant goals are sought.
- Adequate controls are in place.
- Samples are selected randomly.
- Measurements are made blindly and without bias.
- Appropriate statistical analysis is applied.

Following these guidelines, we can develop a checklist for reviewing a trial protocol:

Overall:

- Statement of objective(s)
- Statement of hypotheses in relation to the objectives

    (It is important to clearly convey the two items above, otherwise the results of the research would be regarded as exploratory, hypothesis generating, or a "fishing expedition.")

- Background, often presented as a literature review
- Rationale for the trial that defines its significance

    (Explain why the research question follows logically from previous research in the literature. Identify specific gaps that the clinical trial is intended to fill.)

- Pharmaceutical information, including source of agents, in the event that agents are to be used

Design Aspects:

- Type of control, randomization, stratification, and degree of blinding.
- Patient eligibility criteria. Must include the disease risk and relevant population characteristics, disease stage, medical history, and prior and concomitant therapies for inclusion and exclusion.
- Sample size requirement and justification. Projection of recruitment period and location of centers require realistic expectations of accrual, effect size, and feasibility.
- Endpoint specification.

    (Prioritize the primary, secondary, and other endpoints. They should correspond to the hypotheses and must address the objectives.)

- Diagnostic criteria.

    (This element relates the disease, condition, or risk and its stage/severity under study. Every study should use the current diagnostic methodology available to all the investigators.)

- Measurement reliability.

    (Measurement reliability helps with interpretation of the study results. The meaningful effect of a treatment needs to be judged against the measurement error.)

- Quality control or quality assurance procedures.

    (Operational procedures for assuring the quality and consistency of the data are important and particularly important to a multicenter trial.)

Conduct Aspects:

- Define timeline for pretreatment evaluation (screening), start of study (baseline), follow-up visits, and end of study

  (Length of follow-up should consider disease severity, assumptions of intervention effect on disease, and time necessary for treatment to work or reach the specified endpoint. These considerations should be balanced with the chance of subjects' withdrawal if the study is too long and the chance that the concept under study will become outdated.)

- Study parameters, lab tests, and patient monitoring

- Frequency, timing, and types of contact with the patient and provisions for long-term follow-up if pertinent to study questions or aims

  (Examples include periodic clinic visits, patients' diary entries or interviews with caretakers, and phone calls.)

- Instructions for treatment administration, dose modification, interruption, rescue medication, and discontinuation of study treatment in case of toxicity or intolerability as determined by patient or by the clinician acting in the best interests of patient safety

- Toxicity monitoring and adverse event reporting

- Treatment evaluation and criteria

- Data collection, record keeping, and data processing

  (For multicenter studies, it is advantageous to have a central laboratory facility for newer tests and methods, to avoid interlab variation and to standardize normal ranges.)

- Statistical methods

  (Includes proper control of type I error/false positive rate, adequate power for primary and key secondary endpoints, considerations of subgroups, trial monitoring, interim assessments, missing data issue, and so on.)

- Human subject protection

  (Approval by an IRB and with ongoing approvals as required.)

- Bibliography

- Appendix

  (Include informed consent form, endpoint evaluation criteria, toxicity criteria, and other procedure references.)

When reviewing a published clinical trial report, in addition to the items listed above, we should pay attention to the following:

- Any exclusions after randomization

- Comparability of baseline characteristics among treatment or comparator groups

- Compliance or adherence to the treatment course
- Appropriate statistical analyses
- Appropriate data summaries and graphical displays
- Major findings in efficacy and safety
- Clear statement of conclusions
- Complete discussion, including possible limitations of the study and suggestions for future research
- In the case of "negative" results, an assessment of alternative hypotheses or obstacles (pitfalls) in the conduct of the study

1.3 Ethics and Safety First

Because clinical trials involve experimentation on human subjects, they prompt ethical and safety concerns. At the beginning of this textbook, students are required to complete an online training program on studies involving human subjects and to obtain a certificate as their first homework exercise; many use the CITI training program. CITI stands for Collaborative Institutional Training Initiative (https://www.citiprogram. org/). This program consists of a series of topics that provide up-to-date regulatory requirements for the protection of human subjects in research (Homework 1.2). These regulatory requirements are the natural outgrowth of historical clinical studies that are today considered unethical, inappropriate, or abusive in their disregard of basic human rights and justice. Consider the problems posed by the blood "transfusion" by month to Pope Innocent VIII in the fifteenth century or, in modern times, the human experimentation on prisoners (and racial "undesirables") by the Nazis, the Tuskegee experiments on the natural behavior of syphilis (in minorities), and the Willowbrook experiments on the transmission of hepatitis in children with intellectual disabilities. As an exercise, pose the rationale for these studies and state why they were inappropriate. These and other such experiments led to several documents to define conduct in clinical studies. In the following sections, we briefly review the important points of some of the historical documents that led into the current regulations for conducting clinical trials.

1.3.1 Nuremberg Code (1947) and Helsinki Declaration (1964)

The Nuremberg Code was established after World War II. Later, the World Medical Association (WMA) published the Helsinki Declaration, which is currently being followed and updated by the WMA. These documents together specify the following ethical principles and guidelines for clinical trials:

- Competent and voluntary consent must be obtained from all participants.
- There should be no reasonable alternative to conducting the experiment (to show the effect of the intervention).
- Study should have a basis in biological knowledge and animal studies.
- Unnecessary suffering and injury must be avoided.
- Participants should have no expectation for death or disability (as a result of participation in the study).
- Any risk should be consistent with the humanitarian importance of the study.
- Study must be conducted by qualified individuals.
- Participants can withdraw, at will, at any time.
- Investigator is under obligation to terminate the experiment if injury seems likely.

1.3.2 Belmont Report (1976)

The Belmont Report provides a more modern perspective to the ethical principles and guidelines.

Respect for Persons
As an application of the principle of respect for persons, IRBs composed of representatives from the fields of science, statistics, ethics, and law, as well as a lay person, are formed to provide ethical oversight of clinical studies at the site of individual investigators. An IRB must approve each protocol before any study can be conducted in that institution. All participants' privacy should be respected and protected.

Beneficence
As an application of the principle of beneficence, the researcher should maximize benefits and minimize risks for trial participants and should make participants cognizant of the potential risks and benefits.

Justice
As an application of the principle of justice, participants should be selected equitably, without exploitation of vulnerable populations. Direct or indirect coercion should be avoided.

For more on the requirements for informed consent, see Temple Health's toolkit, *A Practical Guide to Informed Consent.**

---

* Temple Health's toolkit. "A Practical Guide to Informed Consent," available from http://www.templehealth.org/ICTOOLKIT/html/ictoolkitpage5.html (accessed on April 5, 2014).

A list of mandatory topics to be included in an informed consent form is given in Appendix 1.1.

The FDA recently issued a draft guidance titled *Informed Consent Information Sheet.* This guidance describes the basic and additional elements of informed consent and includes topics such as review of patient records, children as subjects, and subject participation in more than one study.

1.3.3 Discussion

"Subject," "participant," "patient," and "volunteer" are common nomenclatures that are often used interchangeably in clinical trials to refer to an individual enrolled in the study. It is interesting to read the ethical principles in the Belmont Report, in which the participants of clinical trials are considered volunteers, and participation in clinical trials is considered a human right that needs to be equitably offered to all eligible persons. First, it is important to recognize that any medical practice based on unproven treatments is likely not ethical. A clinical trial is ethical when there is adequate collective doubt about the value of the new therapy (Fredrickson 1968) or a suggestion that another treatment or approach may be superior. Therefore, a clinical trial is a necessary step as an investigation for advancing medical practice in both efficacy and safety. In some parts of the world, newspapers occasionally have shocking headlines such as "Drug Testing on Our School Children," "Deaths and Injuries in Drug Trial," "Patients Treated with Sugar Pills," etc. Without understanding the details, readers often gain a misleading picture of clinical trials from these eye-catching titles. Those who study the doctrines of appropriate clinical trial design and conduct will hopefully be inspired to educate others, whenever there is an opportunity to do so, about the correct concept and method of clinical trials. Secondly, as citizens of the society and also consumers of medical products, the public needs to understand the FDA and other regulatory agencies' responsibility to approve medicines and devices to protect the public health.

Ethical considerations also have a strong impact on such aspects of study design as randomization, blinding, placebo control, sequential design for monitoring safety and efficacy, early stopping procedures, etc. Subjects' right to withdraw and investigators' obligation to remove any endangered subject from participation in a trial have also led to the ubiquitous problem of missing data in clinical trials. Chapter 10 is devoted to dealing with the issue of missing data.

---

* US Department of Health and Human Services, Food and Drug Administration, OGCP, CDER, CBER, CDRH (2014). "Informed Consent Information Sheet: Guidance for IRBs, Clinical Investigators, and Sponsors," available from http://www.fda.gov/RegulatoryInformation/Guidances/ucm101975.htm (accessed on July 21, 2014).

In summary, all fundamental issues in clinical trials can be viewed as arising from the need to balance rigorous scientific experimentation with ethical medical practice. For a good scientific experiment, we expect the clinical trial to provide valid and efficient answers to the hypothesis being tested. On the other hand, we also require that the clinical trial be designed and conducted realistically to follow good medical practice. The feasibility of conducting a clinical trial is the key to its success. Statistics provides scientific validity and efficiency, whereas laws, rules, regulations, and oversight uphold ethics.

1.4 Classifications of Clinical Trials

In the study and discussion of clinical trials, we often come across different descriptions for trials in the literature. Because different types of trials may lead to different issues and require different methods for analysis, it is useful to make classifications as follows.

1.4.1 By Medical Intervention

For example:

- Drug
- Biologic (e.g., vaccine)
- Surgical, radiological procedures
- Medical device
- Screening approaches and technologies
- Behavior modification to achieve health goals
- Biomarker assessments

Note that the FDA's different branches (CDER, CBER, CDRH) are set up to review these interventions.*

1.4.2 By Disease or Therapeutic Area

For example:

- Oncology
- Cardiovascular—heart, lung, blood

---

* CDER—Center for Drug Evaluation and Research; CBER—Center for Biologics Evaluation and Research; CDRH—Center for Devices and Radiological Health.

- Infectious diseases (e.g., HIV/AIDS)
- Neurological, psychological disorders
- Endocrine diseases (e.g., diabetes, osteoporosis)
- Renal and metabolic disorders
- Mental health disorders

Note that each of these areas corresponds to an area of research at one of the institutes at the NIH.

1.4.3 By the Phase of Drug Development as the Stage of the Experiment

Most of the clinical trials on drugs are classified according to whether they take place before (Phases 0[*], I, II, and III) or after (Phase IV) an NDA is sent to the FDA. The trial phases are sequentially numbered from early to late phases in the development of therapeutic agents. In many ways, the earlier the trial phase, the closer the design approaches an ideal experiment in that experimental conditions, such as objectives, participants, and doses, are more restrictive and well controlled. The study duration is relatively shorter and the goals of the study can be accomplished with a smaller sample (enrolled subject) size. Objective measurements are often the endpoints, and safety is the driving concern. By contrast, the later phase studies often recruit a study population closer to a generalized target population reflecting medical practice with realistic complications, resulting in less restriction on the study design. The sample size is relatively larger and the study duration is usually much longer. Subjective clinical endpoints are often preferred. For example, survival duration is a well-defined and measurable endpoint used in many later phase studies (and considered the "gold standard"). The early phases, as weighing more on scientific experiments, tend to be exploratory in nature and often confirm biological principles. The later phases are confirmatory for defined endpoints of clinical benefit for regulatory approval of the efficacy and still, to a certain extent, an expansion of the safety profile of the drug under investigation. Phase III trials are usually considered a high level of evidence and thus are often pivotal to regulatory approval to market the medical product. A recent development, further discussed later, is the accelerated approval process from earlier phase studies when clinical efficacy is seen in an area with a paucity of treatments (unmet medical need), but these approvals often come with a commitment to complete an appropriate later (Phase III) trial. Pharmaceutical and biotech companies usually prepare a comprehensive medical study plan that includes all trials to be conducted in their drug development process with target timelines. This scheme may not be appropriate for trials conducted in an academic setting.

---

[*] For definition of phase 0 trial see Coloma PM (2013) and CDER (2006).

Scheme of Phases of Clinical Trials in Drug Development Process (Non-Oncology)

Ideal Experiment (With Restrictive Conditions)		Real-Life Practice (With Complications)	
Phase I	Phase II	Phase III	Phase IV
Subjects Condition:			
Healthy	Mild disease	Moderate to severe disease	All stages
Main Goals:			
Dose finding Safety response	Early efficacy and safety	Confirmatory efficacy and limited safety	Long-term follow-up safety and efficacy
Bioavailability (absorption, metabolism distribution, elimination)			
Clinical pharmacology			
Major Design:			
Crossover design		Parallel groups design	
Sample Size Range:			
$n = 20$–40		n in the hundreds per group	

It should be noted that the scheme for oncology trials is very different from that above. Because cancer is a devastating disease, patients in Phase I oncology trials are usually in those who have received previous treatments and exhausted potentially effective options. An exception would be for an individual with a cancer for which there is no known effective therapy. The main aims of such trials are to define the optimal dose for further testing, defining safety and toxicity, and exploration of the pharmacokinetics (what the body does to the drug) and pharmaco-dynamics (what the drug does to the body). With recent advances in bio-marker research as exemplified in genomic research, cancer therapies for specific targets have become popular in clinical trials. These trials involve screening and diagnosis of particular groups of cancer patients carry-ing specific gene mutations. Phase I trials that match a target gene muta-tion with the targeting agent for that mutation have shown considerable promise, as illustrated by Tsimberidou et al. (2012). Phase II cancer trials, designed to better calibrate clinical benefit (such as objective response rate and progression-free survival), are often completed in a shorter timeframe and include a smaller sample size compared to Phase III studies. Usually tumor shrinkage is used as the primary endpoint and *progression-free survival* (PFS) as the secondary endpoint. Phase III cancer trials often use PFS or ideally, the *overall survival* (OS), that is, counting deaths from all causes as events, as the primary endpoint. However, as noted above, other less objectively measured endpoints have entered into this arena of trials.

Considering the rising cost of drug development in terms of economical parameters and human suffering from disease, many investigators, trial sponsors, and regulatory agencies are pursuing strategies for shortening the development process. For example, modifying study design to seamlessly combine some of the trial phases might eliminate the time needed for recruiting new centers and initiating another round of grant reviews, contracts, and IRB approvals. Whether this approach actually saves any of the time or cost of drug development remains to be seen, but related statistical issues in these trials, especially in controlling the overall type I error rate, have already been and are currently being investigated by many researchers.

For the regulatory authority to expedite the NDA review process, two important documents are the 1997 FDA Modernization Act, Section 112, entitled *Expediting Study and Approval of Fast Track Drugs* ("the Act") and the FDA's *Guidance for Industry: Fast Track Drug Development Programs* (FTDDP), FDA (2014). The purpose of the FTDDP is to facilitate the development and expedite the review of new drugs that are intended to treat serious or life-threatening conditions and that demonstrate the potential to address unmet medical needs. The Act states that an application for approval of a fast track product may be approved if it is determined that "the product has an effect on a clinical endpoint or on a surrogate endpoint that is reasonably likely to predict clinical benefit." However, the Act also puts limitations on accelerated approval: the sponsor must conduct appropriate postapproval (Phase III or IV) studies to validate the surrogate endpoint or otherwise confirm the effect on the clinical endpoint. The FDA may also withdraw approval of a fast track product using expedited procedures if, among other concerns such as safety issues, the sponsor fails to conduct the required study or if a postapproval study of the fast track product fails to verify the clinical benefit of the product. For example, IRESSA™ (gefitinib tablets 250 mg) was approved under the accelerated approval regulation as monotherapy for the treatment of patients with locally advanced or metastatic non-small cell lung cancer (NSCLC) after failure of both platinum-based and docetaxel chemotherapies in May 2003. The effectiveness of IRESSA was initially based on *objective response rates* (ORR). Subsequent studies intended to demonstrate an increase in survival have been unsuccessful. IRESSA's claim for NSCLC treatment was removed in June 2005 (Drugs@FDA, 2005). Thus, accelerated approval is only conditional approval for a drug. Nevertheless, the prospect of early availability on the market of a drug has broad implications for patients as well as for the drug manufacturer. A recent study (Moore and Furberg 2013) reported that eight drugs approved in 2008 under FTDDP took a median of 5.1 years of clinical development time to gain approval, compared with 7.5 years for 12 drugs under standard review. A striking example of this accelerated approval is seen in the drug Xalkori® (crizotinib capsules), where conditional, accelerated approval was granted in August 2011 based on durable

ORR in two single-arm open-label studies (NCI, 2013). In November 2013, the FDA granted regular approval for crizotinib for the treatment of patients with metastatic NSCLC based on an open-label active-controlled multinational randomized trial (with 347 patients enrolled). In this trial, crizotinib demonstrated superior PFS and ORR in patients with anaplastic lymphoma kinase (ALK)–positive NSCLC whose disease progressed after platinum-based doublet chemotherapy. Accelerated approval has also stimulated the pharmaceutical industry to explore other approaches to improve trial efficiency. However, because fewer patients are studied as part of the expedited drug approval process, such drugs may reach the market with significant safety questions unanswered. The statistical issues surrounding two kinds of type I errors, namely, the "conditional approval" and "final approval" type I errors, are discussed in the study by Shih et al. (2003).

In addition to the major phases in the above scheme, there are Phase 0 and Phase V clinical trials. Phase 0 trials are exploratory IND studies that involve very limited human exposure and usually have no therapeutic or diagnostic intent. Phase 0 trials bridge the gap between traditional preclinical testing and clinical studies; these trials are intended to provide a better understanding of a new compound's pharmacokinetics (PKs), pharmacodynamics (PDs), organ penetration, and effect on the putative target of the intervention before the initiation of Phase I trials. These Phase 0 trials often compare preoperative biopsies with surgically excised tissue following short exposure to the agent in question and thus pose unique statistical and ethical questions. Phase V trials are studies conducted following NDA approval in order to seek additional marketing claims for new indications, sometimes with new formulations or combinations with other approved compounds. Because the compound was already approved for another indication earlier, some previous safety, PK, PD, and dose-ranging information might be able to be used and may not need to be repeated for the new claim application.

1.4.4 By Disease Present (Remedial/Therapeutic Trials) or Absent (Prevention Trials)

Prevention trials can further be classified into *primary* or *secondary prevention*. Primary prevention seeks to intervene in the processes that induce the disease by either lifestyle modifications (changing destructive habits) or by therapeutic agents of very low toxicity intended to disrupt the carcinogenic process. For example, vaccine trials are often primary prevention as are smoking cessation trials, which typify a lifestyle behavior modification approach. Secondary prevention trials often appear as early diagnosis trials (such as screening studies) or as intervention trials, since the objective is to prevent recurrence or postpone further progression of the disease. For example, the National Lung Screening Trial (NLST) was a secondary prevention trial that compared chest X-rays (previously shown as not especially helpful) with low-dose CT scans, the latter of which reduced lung cancer specific mortality by nearly 20% in an at-risk population by finding disease at an earlier stage (National Lung Screening Trial Research Team 2011). The landmark Simvastatin Scandinavian Survival Study (also known as the 4S study) was a secondary prevention study that was designed to evaluate the effect of a cholesterol-lowering drug called simvastatin on mortality and morbidity in patients with coronary heart disease.

In general, all prevention trials are held to much higher safety standards by the IRB and other regulatory agencies because participants are either healthy or have lower disease severity. In addition, prevention trials often require longer study time and larger sample sizes, especially when the incidence rate of the primary clinical endpoint is low for relatively healthier participants. The possibility of using surrogate endpoints (e.g., antibody counts in vaccine trials) is an important design consideration, and the identification of appropriate biomarkers is a strong necessity.

Further reading regarding the design of prevention trials can be found in Shih and Wang (1991) (Homework 1.3).

1.4.5 By Design Feature

- Single site or multicenter
- Placebo, concurrent active control, or historical control
- Crossover or parallel groups
- Fixed dose or titrated dose
- Fixed sample size or group sequential design
- Open label or blind (single, double, or triple blind)
- Number of arms
- Geographical extent (local, regional, or global)

1.4.6 By Hypothesis and Statistical Inference

- Exploratory (hypothesis-generating) trial
- Superiority trial
- Proof of comparability (equivalence or noninferiority trial)

1.5 Multidisciplinary Teamwork in Clinical Trials

To conclude this chapter, we emphasize that clinical trials, as an enterprise, require organization and teamwork. All members of the team must recognize the specialties of the team members and their contributions to the study to facilitate collaboration and thus a successful trial. Functional personnel in a clinical trial team may consist of the following:

- Scientists, including biochemists, biologists, toxicologists, pharmacologists, and biomarker specialists
- Medical monitor and project coordinator
- Clinical investigators and pharmacists at hospitals and medical centers
- Specialists in data management, quality assurance, computer technology
- Statistician and epidemiologist
- Regulatory affairs staff
- Chemical engineer and drug-supply manager
- Marketing personnel
- Bioethicist, patient advocate, voluntary participants

Appendix 1.1: Elements of Informed Consent

The informed consent discussion, written informed consent form, and any other written information to be provided to participants of a trial should include explanations of the following mandatory topics:

1. That the study involves research.
2. The purpose of the study and approximate number of subjects involved in the study.
3. The expected duration of the subject's participation in the study.
4. The study treatment(s) and the probability for random assignment to each treatment.
5. The study procedures to be followed, including all invasive procedures.
6. Those aspects of the study that are experimental.
7. The reasonably foreseeable risks or inconveniences to the subject and, when applicable, to an embryo, fetus, or nursing infant.
8. The reasonably expected benefits. When there is no intended clinical benefit to the subject, the subject should be made aware of this.
9. The alternative procedure(s) or course(s) of treatment that may be available to the subject and their important potential benefits and risks.

10. The records identifying the subject will be kept confidential and, to the extent permitted by the applicable laws and/or regulations, will not be made publicly available. If the results of the study are published, the subject's identity will remain confidential.

11. That the study sponsor, monitor and/or their representative, the IRB/IEC, and the regulatory authority(ies) will be granted direct access to the subject's original medical records for verification of clinical study procedures and/or data, without violating the confidentiality of the subject, to the extent permitted by the applicable laws and regulations and that, by signing and dating a written informed consent form, the subject or the subject's legally acceptable representative is authorizing such access.*

12. The subject's responsibilities.

13. The compensation and/or treatment available to the subject in the event of study-related injury.

14. The anticipated prorated payment, if any, to the subject for participating in the study.

15. The person(s) to contact for further information regarding the study and the rights of study subjects and whom to contact in the event of study-related injury.

16. That the subject's participation in the trial is voluntary and that the subject may refuse to participate or withdraw from the study, at any time, without penalty or loss of benefits to which the subject is otherwise entitled.

17. The foreseeable circumstances and/or reasons under which the subject's participation in the study may be terminated.

18. The anticipated expenses, if any, that subject will incur as a result of participation in the study.

19. The consequences of a subject's decision to withdraw from the research and procedures for orderly termination of participation by the subject.

20. That the subject or the subject's legally acceptable representative will be informed in a timely manner if information becomes available that may be relevant to the subject's willingness to continue participation in the study.

21. Any element(s) required by local regulations (e.g., FDA, other non-US health authorities).

---

* Institutional ethics committee.

The following additional topics are mandatory for inclusion in the informed consent of studies enrolling women of childbearing potential (WOCBP):

1. General Statement

    The subject must not be pregnant and should not become pregnant during exposure to the investigational product unless that is the endpoint of the study. Subjects should be instructed to contact the investigator if they plan to change their contraception method or if they need to take any prescription drug or other medication not prescribed by investigator. Sexually active subjects must use an effective method of contraception during the course of the study, in a manner such that risk of failure is minimized. The informed consent must indicate that information on pregnancy prevention for WOCBP has been reviewed with the subject by the investigator or study designee.

2. Laboratory and Animal Reproductive Toxicology

    The consent should include a statement addressing what is known about the investigational product from laboratory and animal reproductive toxicity studies concerning possible mutagenic and/or teratogenic effects. The consent should indicate that this information has limited predictive value for humans.

3. Unforeseeable Risks

    The consent must indicate that exposure to the investigational product may involve currently unforeseeable risks to the subject (or embryo or fetus, if the subject is or may become pregnant).

4. Occurrence of Pregnancy or Suspected Pregnancy

    The informed consent must include study contact name(s) and telephone number(s) for the subject to call if she becomes pregnant or suspects pregnancy, has missed her period or it is late, or if she has a change in her usual menstrual cycle (e.g., heavier bleeding during her period or bleeding between periods).

5. Discontinuation from the Study

    Any subject who becomes pregnant during the course of the study will be immediately withdrawn (unless allowed or stated differently in the protocol) and referred for obstetrical care. All financial aspects of obstetrical, child, or related care are the responsibility of the subject.

6. Pregnancy Follow-Up

    If a subject becomes pregnant, the investigator will seek access to the subject's and/or infant's clinic/hospital records through the pregnancy, and for a minimum of 8 weeks following delivery.

7. Use of a Study-Prohibited Contraceptive Method

When applicable, the informed consent should clearly indicate if a contraceptive method is prohibited (e.g., when hormonal contraceptive interaction with the investigational product(s) is known or suspected). In this situation, a study participant should be instructed to notify the investigator or study designee if a prohibited contraceptive method is initiated during the course of the study so that additional precautions can be taken or the subject discontinued from the study.

8. Noninvestigational Product Interactions with Hormonal Contraceptives

Women using a hormonal method of contraceptive (e.g., oral contraceptives or implantable or injectable agents) must be instructed to notify the investigator or study designee of the need to take any prescription drug or other medication not prescribed by the investigator. The purpose of this statement is to identify any potential noninvestigational product interaction with the contraceptive that might reduce the effectiveness of the contraceptive method.

Sources: *Protocol under US IND number and/or non-IND: 40710 (Feb-05-1999). A multicenter, double-blind, placebo-controlled, randomized fixed-dose study of nefazodone ER in the treatment of depressed patients.*

Homework 1.1

The following are excerpts from three LOIs produced by a university cancer center in a training course. Suppose that you are a reviewer and have been asked to provide critiques and constructive suggestions to the researchers. Based on your learning of the course so far, comment on each of them regarding the following aspects: (a) Is the proposed study a clinical trial? Why or why not? (b) Are the study objective(s) clearly stated? (c) Does the design (including the endpoints and statistical consideration) match the objective? If not, provide suggestion(s).

LOI – 1

**Use of the Memorial Symptom Assessment
Scale in Patients with Cervical Cancer**

Objectives
Determine the intensity of symptoms and the distress those symptoms cause in patients with cervical cancer.

The Rationale for Performing the Trial
There is currently a lack of literature regarding the use of the Memorial Symptom Assessment Scale in cervical cancer. Determining the symptoms experienced by women who have cervical cancer will be helpful in the further elucidation of interventions to alleviate these symptoms. Further study would also assist in determining the impact of these symptoms on patients' quality of life and their ability to function as women.

Design would be Used to Accomplish the Main Objectives of the Trial
Use of questionnaires and description of independent variables with correlation statistics to determine significance.

LOI – 2

Study of Safety and Effectiveness of the Use of Gemcitabine and Irinotecan in Women with Refractory Ovarian Cancer

Objectives
1. The primary objective is to determine toxicity and response to combination therapy with irinotecan and gemcitabine in refractory ovarian cancer.
2. Secondary objectives are to estimate the time to progression and median survival time.
3. An exploratory objective is to assess whether there is a correlation between response and P-gp and CD44 expression in the original tumor and/or recurrent tumor.

Rationale
Irinotecan and gemcitabine are well-tolerated single agents, each with ovarian cancer antitumor activity. Combining the two agents is appealing because each has a potentially distinct mechanism of action. Irinotecan inhibits topoisomerase I and gemcitabine inhibits DNA polymerases by competing with dCTP for the enzymes. Gemcitabine also serves as a substrate for polymerases by competing with dCTP for the enzymes and as a substrate for polymerase ε and polymerase α by further inhibiting DNA synthesis. Furthermore, irinotecan stabilizes DNA strands that offers sites for insertion of gemcitabine triphosphate during relegation of DNA. Preclinical data suggests dose-dependent synergistic interactions for the two drugs in lung small cell cancer, breast cancer, and HL-60 leukemia cell lines. Maximum tolerated dose for the gemcitabine/irinotecan combination was determined in a Phase I study. This study was followed by a Phase II trial testing this combination in pancreatic cancer and showed some efficacy. Although combination regimens using gemcitabine have been explored in the treatment of ovarian cancer, the gemcitabine/irinotecan combination has never been tested.

In ovarian cancer, second-line regimens usually involve single-drug therapy. These regimens have only limited response (17–30%) of short duration (median response 4 months). Better regimens using drug combination are needed.

Our laboratory has data that suggests a possible correlation between ovarian cancer expression of CD44 and drug resistance. We also have preliminary data correlating CD44 expression and P-gp expression in resistant ovarian cancer cells. There is also published data correlating CD44 expression in breast cancer with P-gp expression. Dr. Smith's laboratory published observations indicating that leukemic cells with high P-gp protein content become more metastatic in vivo when treated with P-gp substrate drugs. These observations suggest that P-gp and CD44 may interact and convey an invasive chemo-resistant phenotype to cancer cells. We are interested in determining the level of expression of these two membrane proteins in recurrent ovarian tumors and correlating these findings with treatment outcome.

If this drug regimen improves 6-month survival, we will then compare this regimen with standard therapy in a Phase III trial.

Study Design
This is a Phase II study of combination therapy with gemcitabine 1000 mg/m^2 (Day 1 and 8) and irinotecan 100 mg/m^2 (Day 1 and 8) every three weeks. Patients diagnosed with recurrent ovarian carcinoma resistant to platinum and good performance status will be eligible. Patients who have received two prior chemotherapy regimens will be eligible. The primary endpoint will be 6 month survival. Secondary endpoints are to estimate time to progression and determine whether there is a correlation between clinical response and tumor CD44 and P-gp levels.

LOI – 3

Ovarian Preservation in Women Undergoing Cancer Therapy

Background
Although cancer therapy has led to marked improvements in disease-free intervals and OS in patients with malignancies, quality of life issues have become a major concern for patients and the physicians caring for them. Many of our therapies lead to ovarian failure in our younger patients due to either high-dose chemotherapy or radiation therapy, leading to the development of menopausal symptoms and loss of fertility. Reproductive endocrinologic techniques are improving, and we can now consider offering our patients ovarian transplantation in a research setting as an alternative to ovarian failure, thus providing the possibility of reestablishing reproductive potential in the future and hopefully leading to an improvement in patients' quality of life.

As in vitro fertilization (IVF) techniques have improved, embryo cryopreservation has become a safe and accepted method of storing the fertilized gamete. The development of technology to cryopreserve unfertilized female gametes has been less successful. There have only been a few pregnancies that have resulted from frozen gametes; this low fertilization rate is a result of hardening of the zona pellucida, an increased incidence of aneuploidy, and damage to the cytoskeleton, leading to significant changes in the organization and trafficking of molecules and organelles. Ovarian cryopreservation has therefore been considered a viable alternative to the cryopreservation of oocytes. Cryopreservation of primoidal follicles found in ovarian tissue has met with greater success, because these follicles are less differentiated, possess fewer organelles, and lack a zona pellucida.

Primordial follicles have been successfully harvested from mice, cryopreserved, and transplanted back into oophorectomized animals. Estrogenic activity and live-born young have been reported after continuous culture of mouse follicles from the primordial stage (1,2)*.

Oktay reported on two patients who underwent ovarian transplantation prior to undergoing surgery or radiation therapy for benign ovarian cysts and Stage IIIB squamous cell carcinoma of the cervix, respectively (3)*. In both patients, menopause was confirmed after transplantation by measuring serum follicle-stimulating hormone. In both patients, restoration of estradiol levels confirmed that the ovaries were functioning, and the patient who underwent surgery for benign ovarian cysts resumed spontaneous ovarian function after transplantation was performed (4)....* Three of the four patients had evidence of resumption of ovarian function, although short-lived. The women involved in the study were 46 to 49 years old, which most likely impacted the reported outcomes. These two case reports provide evidence that this is a viable treatment option we can begin to offer our patients in a research setting.

Trial Design
This will be a prospective trial consisting of several tiers. Eligibility criteria will include the following:

1. Age of diagnosis (less than 40)
2. Menstrual status (premenopausal) based on markers including follicle-stimulating hormone (FSH), estradiol, and inhibin, as well as a transvaginal ultrasound
3. Desire to preserve ovarian function for fertility reasons or to prevent the development of menopause
4. Treatment regimen consisting of chemotherapy, radiation therapy, or a combination that will most likely render the patient sterile at the completion of their treatment

---

* Four citations and a treatment schema in the original LOI are omitted here.

When a patient is identified, she will be approached to determine if she is interested in ovarian transplantation. If she declines, she will be asked to participate in our quality of life questionnaire to determine if there is an improvement in the quality of life of the patients receiving ovarian transplantation versus the patients who do not.

Patients who agree to participate will then enter the treatment portion of the trial, which will consist of trying to prevent ovarian failure through the use of GnRH agonists or antagonists prior to chemotherapy or radiation therapy. Women whose normal ovarian function is maintained will enter the quality of life component of the study and be followed regarding future pregnancy outcomes and the development of menopause. Women who unfortunately develop ovarian failure will undergo transplantation of ovarian tissue. These patients will be followed for resumption of menstrual function and pregnancy outcomes. A treatment schema is attached.

Objectives
1. Successful transplantation of ovarian tissue with resumption of ovarian function, reversal of menopausal symptoms, and restoration of reproductive function
2. Determine whether GnRH agonists or GnRH antagonists are better at preserving ovarian function in women receiving chemotherapy or radiation therapy
3. Determine if the quality of life of patients participating in the clinical trial is improved compared to that of patients who decline to participate
4. Determine prognostic factors of ovarian recovery in women receiving chemotherapy (both epidemiologic and molecular markers)

Homework 1.2

Log in to https://www.citiprogram.org/ and complete the in-depth training on the protection of human subjects in research. Obtain a certificate of completion for the CITI program.

Homework 1.3

Reading: "Overview of Some Important Issues in Designing Clinical Trials for Prevention of Chronic Diseases" (Shih, W. J., and Wang, C., *Pharmaceutical Medicine* 1991, 5: 87–96).

References

Baumgardner KR. (1997). A review of key research design and statistical analysis issues. *Journal of Oral Surgery, Oral Medicine, Oral Pathology, Oral Radiology, and Endodontics* 84: 550–556.

Burns PB, Rohrich RJ, and Chung KC. (2011). The levels of evidence and their role in evidence-based medicine. *Plastic and Reconstructive Surgery* 128: 305–310.

CDER (Center for Drug Evaluation and Research). Guidance for Industry, Investigators, and Reviewers: Exploratory IND Studies (2006). http://www.fda.gov/downloads/Drugs/GuidanceComplianceRegulatoryInfomration/Guidance//ucm078933.pdf (accessed April 5, 2014).

Coloma PM. (2013). Phase 0 clinical trials: Theoretical and practical implications in oncologic drug development. *Open Access Journal of Clinical Trials* 5: 119–126.

Cramer DW. (1974). The role of cervical cytology in the declining morbidity and mortality of cervical cancer. *Cancer* 34: 2018–2027.

Ederer F. (1979). The statistician's role in developing a protocol for a clinical trial. *The American Statistician* 33: 116–119.

FDA (US Food and Drug Administration). Speeding Access to Important New Therapies: Fast Track, Accelerated Approval and Priority Review. www.fda.gov/forconsumers/byaudience/forpatientadvocates/speedingaccesstoimportantnewtherapies/ucm128291.htm (accessed April 5, 2014).

FDA (US Food and Drug Administration). (2004). Challenge and Opportunity on the Critical Path to New Medical Products. http://www.fda.gov/downloads/ScienceResearch/SpecialTopics/ClinicalPathInitiative/CriticalPathOpportunitiesReports/ucm113411.pdf (accessed April 5, 2014).

FDA. Code for Federal Regulations, Title 21, Part 50. Protection of Human Subjects. http://www.accessdata.fda.gov/scripts/cdrh/cfdocs/cfcfr/CFRsearch.cfm?CFRPart=50 (accessed April 5, 2014).

Fredrickson DS. (1968). The field trial: Some thoughts on the independent ordeal. *Bulletin of the New York Academy of Medicine* 44: 985–993.

Friedman LM, Furberg CD, and DeMets DL. (1996). *Fundamentals of Clinical Trials*. New York: Springer.

Hill AB. (1937). General summary and conclusions. *Lancet* I: 883–885.

Melnyk BM and Fineout-Overholt E. (2010). *Evidence-Based Practice in Nursing and Healthcare: A Guide to Best Practice*. Lippincott, Philadelphia, Williams & Wilkins.

Michael CW. (1999). The Papanicolaou smear and the obstetric patient: A simple test with great benefits. *Diagnostic Cytopathology* 21(1): 1–3.

Moore TJ and Furberg CD. (2013). Development times, clinical testing, postmarket follow-up, and safety risks for the new drugs approved by the US Food and Drug Administration: The class of 2008. *JAMA Internal Medicine* 174: 90–95. doi:10.1001/jamainternmed.2013.11813.

National Cancer Institute. (2013). Cancer Drug Information: FDA Approval for Crizotinib. http://www.cancer.gov/cancertopics/druginfo/fda-crizotinib (accessed April 5, 2014).

National Lung Screening Trial Research Team. (2011). The National Lung Screening Trial: Overview and study design. *Radiology* 258(1): 243–253. doi:10.1148/radiol.10091808.

Shih WJ, Ouyang P, Quan H, Lin Y, Michiels B, and Bijnens L. (2003). Controlling type I error rate for fast track drug development programmes. *Statistics in Medicine* 22: 665–675.

Shih WJ and Wang C. (1991). Overview of some important issues in designing clinical trials for prevention of chronic diseases. *Pharmaceutical Medicine* 5: 87–96.

Tsimberidou AM, Iskander NG, Hong DS, Wheler JJ, Falchook GS, and Fu S. (2012). Personalized medicine in a phase I clinical trials program: the MD Anderson Cancer Center initiative. *Clinical Cancer Research* 18(22): 6373–6383.

2

Concepts and Methods of Statistical Designs

As we mentioned in Chapter 1, most fundamental design issues in clinical trials arise from the need to strike a balance between scientific experiment and good clinical practice in a trial. Whereas laws and regulations guard the ethical aspects of trial design, statistics addresses scientific validity and efficiency, which in turn enhance the medical ethics and practice. Although many design issues surface in the development of a clinical trial, in this chapter we focus on the major concerns for trial validity, and we discuss the concerns for trial efficiency in Chapter 3. First, we consider the various types of validity: external validity, internal validity, and repeatability. We then explore the phenomenon of regression toward the mean to illustrate a kind of bias, which can be accounted for when there is a concurrent control group in the design. Logically, we need to consider at least two observations per subject in a clinical trial, one as the baseline and the other as a follow-up measurement. In this two-dimensional setting, we review the notion of bivariate normal distribution and the expression of simple linear regression as we discuss the topic of regression toward the mean. Finally, we conclude this chapter by discussing several methods of randomization and blinding that are commonly used in clinical trials to make the control group fully functional for achieving internal validity.

2.1 External Validity

External validity is the validity of inferences as they pertain to the generalizability to future subjects rather than the specific trial participants (Rothwell, 2005). It implies the applicability of the study results to general medical practice. Richard Horton (2000), past editor of *The Lancet*, once commented that "the issues of eternal validity are the most important that face clinical research today and that the failure to resolve them is largely responsible for the indifference doctors world wide show toward research evidence." Many agree that this is what *evidence-based medicine* represents: getting research evidence into practice (Evidence-Based Medicine Working Group, 1992). Within the framework of a clinical trial protocol, the characteristics of patients, treatment and procedures, outcome measures, and follow-up in the trial protocol together define the generalizability and applicability of the trial results. For any New Drug Application (NDA), these data are the basis for the information contained in the drug package insert and will greatly influence the "labeled" indications for use and thus the marketing implications for the drug manufacturer. Manufacturers would like to make the product available to the widest possible population; hence, they would prefer the eligibility criteria (defined by the "Inclusion/exclusion criteria" section) to be as loose as possible. By contrast, clinical scientists would like to control the heterogeneity of trial participants to isolate the signal from the noise, thus they would prefer a set of more focused inclusion and exclusion criteria. Because the trial has a better chance of fulfilling its scientific aim when these criteria are more focused, balancing these two needs is a very important consideration in the trial design.

When we consider the patient population included and data generated in a trial, we should recognize that the participants in a clinical trial, at least in concept, represent a sample of all potential participants defined by the inclusion and exclusion criteria of the study protocol. This representativeness allows generalization to future recipients and users of the medical product under investigation. When the study is finished, we can thus assume that the baseline characteristics of the participants in the trial reflect the patient population as defined by the eligibility criteria in the study design. On the other hand, we might also find out that dropouts and missing data occurred, which could cause incomplete information. The path from the target population to which the medical product is to be applied to the actual data samples used for analyses is a *sampling process*. The reverse direction, where we use data analyses to derive conclusions from the sample data for application to the target population, is an *inferential process* (Figure 2.1). Inferences are made based on observed data, statistical methods, and certain assumptions. One such assumption is that the data generated in the trial are derived from a *random* sample of the target population. The extent of the generalizability or applicability of the trial results, that is, the external validity of the trial, depends on how closely this assumption approaches reality.

To evaluate this concept further, let us consider the lipid-lowering treatment for prevention of coronary heart disease (CHD) as an example. The Coronary Drug Project (1973) studied a cholesterol-lowering therapy (Cholestyramine) in men between the ages of 30 and 64 who had experienced at least one myocardial infarction (MI), that is, heart attack. The criteria involving the specific gender, age, and baseline condition (such as prior MIs) of patients limited the generalizability of Cholestyramine's efficacy to a larger population. Almost 20 years later, the 4S study (Simvastatin Scandinavian Survival Study 1994) tested Zocor® and reported a reduction in major coronary events for both sexes, aged 60 or more. This was an astonishing medical advancement in cholesterol-lowering therapy for older individuals of both genders. Nevertheless, the efficacy was indicated only for patients with hypercholesterolemia.

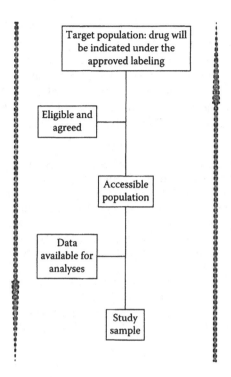

FIGURE 2.1
Sampling path (from top to bottom) and inferential path (reverse direction) for external validity of a clinical trial.

Finally, a primary prevention study of acute coronary events tested Mevacor® in men and women with average cholesterol levels (Downs et al. 1998) and fully extended the efficacy for the class of cholesterol-lowering medicines (HMG-CoA reductase inhibitors) to the general public. Subsequent studies with various HMG-CoA inhibitors resulted in differential FDA labeling (e.g., Crestor®) for MI prevention based on the protocol's patient inclusion and exclusion criteria and endpoints.

In addition to the eligibility criteria, the investigator's medical practice site can also be a factor for the external validity of a clinical trial. In this regard, to extend generalizability, the later phases of a clinical trial should be conducted by multiple investigators in a variety of medical settings, including university teaching hospitals, community medical centers, private clinics, etc., as well as in various geographical regions that may have different environmental and practice conventions. A discrete example of this problem is illustrated by the case of the Serostim® NDA for the treatment of short bowel syndrome. In June of 2003, the FDA Gastrointestinal Drugs Advisory Committee rejected the manufacturer's NDA primarily because of the lack of generalizability of the pivotal study: the study had included only two centers, one of which accrued the vast majority of patients. Only after the manufacturer conducted a further study in more and diverse centers, as requested by the FDA, was the medicine approved for open use and marketing.

Despite the examples above, assessment of external validity can be very complex and usually requires more clinical than statistical expertise. There are no accepted guidelines on how the external validity of randomized clinical trials (RCTs) should be assessed. However, Horton (2000) made a summary of questions asked by Julian and Pocock (1997) as a helpful checklist:

Patients Studied
1. Were the patients included in the trial adequately representative of the patients to be encountered in normal clinical practice? Were the eligibility criteria too narrow or too broad?
2. Were adequate steps taken to ensure that a high proportion of eligible patients was randomized? In particular, was a log kept of all patients with the appropriate condition, and how do randomized patients compare with those not randomized (both eligible and ineligible)?
3. Was the setting of the trial and the manner of patient selection appropriate? Were the eligibility criteria too narrow or too broad? Have the [investigators] inappropriately extrapolated their findings to types of patients that were not adequately represented?

Treatments
1. Was the treatment under comparison, including dose schedule, duration of treatment, non-compliance, and the control regimens (placebo or standard treatment) appropriate for normal clinical practice and determining future treatment policy in such patients?
2. Were all aspects of current good clinical practice (for example, ancillary care) adequately taken into account?

Outcome Measures and Follow-up
1. Were the outcome measures (endpoints, indicators of patient response) appropriate for reaching overall conclusions about the treatments under investigation?
2. Was too much evidence given to surrogate markers of response (for example, physiological indicators) rather than to more major indicators of overall prognosis (for example, mortality, major clinical events)?
3. Was the duration of treatment and length of patient follow-up sufficiently reliable to assess the efficacy and safety of treatment?
4. Were adequate steps taken to elicit all relevant adverse events and side-effects of treatment?

Balanced Discussion and Conclusion
1. Have the authors given adequate considerations to the limitations of their study in all the above respects?

2. Have the authors given a balanced account of evidence from other related studies or have they given undue weight to their own findings?

Source: Horton, R., *Statistics in Medicine*, 19: 3149–3164, 2000. With permission.

2.2 Internal Validity

Internal validity is the reasonable representation of the treatment effects within the study population. Internal validity is a prerequisite for external validity. The primary concerns for internal validity are as follows:

- If differences in the treatment groups are observed, are the differences due to patient characteristics, the treatments, or chance?

  (Logically, the goal for validity here is to rule out patients and chance as causes of the effect.)

- If no differences are observed in the treatment groups, is this fact due to misconduct, lack of precision (study power), or true equivalence?

  (In this case, the goal for validity is to rule out misconduct or lack of power.)

The fundamental idea for supporting internal validity is to design trials that include comparable groups such that the outcomes, whether different or the same, measure only the effect of the treatment, and nothing else. To accomplish this goal, we should adhere to the methodologies below to avoid or minimize bias in the following areas:

- treatment allocation—by use of randomization and stratification
- assessing treatment effects—by use of a concurrent control group and by masking the treatment group assignment
- study monitoring and data analysis—by use of ongoing review by disciplined investigators and expert statisticians
- fishing expeditions—by setting predefined hypotheses and endpoints in the protocol.

2.3 Repeatability

The basic philosophy for repeatability of clinical trials is that scientific experiments should be verified by replication. The FDA usually favors applications with two or more pivotal trials for the approval of an NDA. These trials may vary somewhat in the patient population or control agent used. Therefore, they are usually not strictly exact replicates. In certain situations, however, a single large trial with different centers showing consistent results may also be acceptable, especially for studies with mortality or serious morbidity endpoints, because these types of trials are hard to repeat, especially in the setting of positive results. Showing consistency among centers and predefined subgroups is essential for demonstrating repeatability in the case of a single large trial.

2.4 The Phenomenon of Regression toward the Mean and Importance of a Concurrent Control Group

In Chapter 1 we noted that Friedman, Furberg, and DeMets (1996) restrict their definition of clinical trials to those that are compared against a control group. Although this definition excludes many single-arm early phase trials in oncology funded by NIH and usually conducted by the designated cancer centers or the cancer cooperative groups (unless their definition also meant to include *historical control* or *self-baseline control*), it highlights the importance of a *concurrent control group* for the internal validity of a clinical trial. We further illustrate this point here by examining the phenomenon of regression toward the mean. We raise this topic in this early chapter because we want readers to review the basic method of regression, which is a prerequisite for the level of this book. Regression methodology is used throughout this book, from the study design stage to data analysis later. The material in Chapter 5 ("Analysis of Covariance and Stratified Analysis") requires readers to be familiar with the regression method.

2.4.1 Regression toward the Mean: Definition and Example

Regression toward the mean is a phenomenon that occurs when a second measurement is made only for those individuals with an "extreme" initial measurement. On average, the second measurement tends to be less extreme than the first, even in the absence of any medical intervention. It came from the phrase *regression towards mediocrity*, which was originally coined by Sir Francis Galton (1886) to characterize the tendency for tall parents to produce shorter offspring and vice versa (Bland and Altman 1994). We should recognize this phenomenon because it often occurs in clinical trials when we include patients with high or low measurements at baseline. For example, we study antihypertensive treatments on patients with high blood pressures, cholesterol-lowering therapies on patients with hyperlipidemia, and bone-strengthening medicines on postmenopausal osteoporotic women with low bone-mineral densities.

In-Class Discussion: Figure 2.2a and b shows two illustrations clipped from the article "Effects of Oral Alendronate and Intranasal Salmon Calcitonin on Bone Mass and Biochemical Markers of Bone Turnover in Postmenopausal Women with Osteoporosis" (Adami et al. 1995). This study was a 24-month trial in postmenopausal women with osteoporosis (low bone density). Patients were randomized into four treatment groups: placebo, alendronate 10 mg, alendronate 20 mg, or calcitonin 100 IU. The left panel (Figure 2.2a) shows the mean percent changes ± SE in lumbar spine bone-mineral density (L-spine BMD) at 6, 12, 18, and 24 months. Based on this information, consider the following questions: Why was there an increase in L-spine BMD in the placebo group at month 6? What did that placebo effect represent?

One might suspect that the placebo effect was due to the calcium supplements (500 mg daily) provided to all of the participants in the trial. This guess seems reasonable but, if it is true, why is there no similar placebo effect shown on the right panel for the trochanter BMD at month 6? A more plausible reason for the placebo effect can be found in the participant selection and eligibility section of the paper. The trial required that "[at baseline] each participant have a lumbar spine bone-mineral density >2 SD below the mean for young premenopausal women (<0.99 g/cm^2 for Lunar® densitometers and <0.86 g/cm^2 for Hologic®, Norland®, and Sophos®), while there was no restriction for the trochanter BMD. Thus, regression toward the mean might be what the placebo effect represents in this case. Interestingly, Cummings et al. (2000) published a later article that supports this reasoning.

2.4.2 Effect of Regression toward the Mean as a Form of Bias

Because clinical trials are follow-up studies, there must be at least two observations per subject: the baseline and the follow-up measurements. In this two-dimensional setting, the notion of bivariate distribution is needed. The bivariate normal distribution and the expression of simple linear regression are very helpful when continuous variables are involved. Let random variable X_1 be the baseline measurement for one treatment group, and X_2 be the follow-up measurement for that same group. Assume a bivariate normal distribution for the paired measurements (X_1, X_2), with the mean vector and covariance matrix shown as follows:

$$\begin{pmatrix} X_1 \\ X_2 \end{pmatrix} \sim N\left(\begin{pmatrix} \mu_1 \\ \mu_2 \end{pmatrix}, \begin{pmatrix} \sigma_1^2 & \rho\sigma_1\sigma_2 \\ \rho\sigma_1\sigma_2 & \sigma_2^2 \end{pmatrix} \right)$$

Recall that, in statistical terms, regression is a conditional analysis. This approach addresses the following question: Given what I observe now

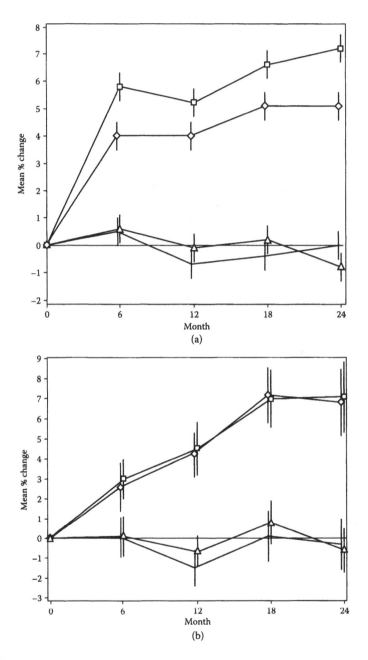

FIGURE 2.2
(a) Lumbar spine bone-mineral density (BMD). Mean percent changes (SE) in BMD with placebo (O), alendronate 10 mg (◊), alendronate 20 mg (□), intranasal salmon calcitonin 100 IU (∇), baseline to 24 months. (b) Trochanter BMD. Mean percent changes (SE) in BMD with placebo (O), alendronate 10 mg (◊), alendronate 20 mg (□), intranasal salmon calcitonin 100 IU (∇), baseline to 24 months. (From Adami S, et al. *Bone,* 17: 383–390, 1995, with permission.)

(at baseline) as X_1, what should I *expect* to see later (at follow-up) as X_2? We can answer this question by using the simple linear regression expression

$$E(X_2|X_1) = \alpha + \beta X_1$$
$$= \mu_2 + \rho\frac{\sigma_2}{\sigma_1}(X_1 - \mu_1) \tag{2.1}$$

where $\alpha = \mu_2 - \beta\mu_1$ and $\beta = \rho\frac{\sigma_2}{\sigma_1}$.

Readers may review the notion of bivariate normal distribution and the simple linear regression expression from an introductory biostatistics textbook (e.g., Daniel 2009).

Assuming no treatment effect in this treatment group (i.e., $\mu_1 = \mu_2 = \mu$ and $\sigma_1 = \sigma_2 = \sigma$), the regression equation can be rewritten for a specific value $X_1 = x_1$ as

$$E(X_2 \mid x_1) = \mu + \rho(x_1 - \mu) \tag{2.2}$$

Subtracting μ from both sides and taking the absolute value, it is clear that the following inequality holds:

$$\left|E(X_2|x_1) - \mu\right| = |\rho| \, |\, x_1 - \mu \,| \le |\, x_1 - \mu \,| \tag{2.3}$$

This inequality tells us that, even with no treatment effect, if the initial value $X_1 = x_1$ is an extreme case (larger or smaller than the population mean μ), the follow-up value X_2 will be, on average, closer to the population mean than x_1. Also known as the "ceiling effect" or "floor effect," the phenomenon of regression toward the mean is a form of bias, that is, no treatment effect seemingly produces an effect!

Equation 2.2 also implies

$$\left| E(X_2|x_1) - x_1 \right| = \left|(\rho - 1) \, (x_1 - \mu)\right| \tag{2.4}$$

This expression says that the magnitude of the effect of regression toward the mean (left-hand side of Equation 2.4) for a specific case $X_1 = x_1$ is usually not zero. It will be zero when $\rho = 1$ (perfect correlation), or if the specific case x_1 is a perfect sample in which it is equal to the population mean μ (Homework 2.1).

In-Class Exercise: Assume that you are conducting a placebo-controlled antihypertensive clinical trial. One of the inclusion criteria says that, in order to be included in the trial, the participant's baseline sitting diastolic blood pressure (SDBP) has to be between 90 to 110 mmHg. Suppose the normal population of the same age group has a mean SDBP of 85 mmHg.

If the correlation between the baseline and follow-up SDBP is 0.5, what would you expect the magnitude of the effect of regression toward the mean to be for participants whose baseline SDBP is 95 mmHg?

Answer: Using Equation 2.4, $|E(X2|X1) - X1| = |(\rho - 1)(X_1 - \mu)| = |0.5 - 1|$ $|95 - 85| = 5 \text{ (mmHg)}$.

2.5 Random Samples and Randomization of Samples

We should distinguish the two kinds of randomness that occur in clinical trials. We should also be sensitive to the perception that a phrase with randomness might imply that the situation is chaotic, without purpose, or out of control to a layman (Featherstone and Donovan 1998). Hence, we should be cautious in our communication.

Randomness as Used Herein: As discussed in Section 2.1 ("External Validity"), consideration of subjects who participate in a clinical trial as conceptually random "samples" is key for generalizing the trial results to the target population in medical practice. This is not the survey-type of sampling, where samples are drawn from a fixed, finite, cross-sectional population. The random samples in clinical trials are conceptually drawn from the current, as well as future, cohorts of users of the medication under study.

When there are two or more interventions in a comparative trial, that is, in a controlled clinical trial, randomization of subjects to treatment groups is a methodology for reaching a certain degree of *internal validity* for the given trial. Random sampling and randomization of samples (subjects) are two distinct types of randomness.

2.5.1 What Is Randomization?

Randomization is a process by which subjects are assigned to treatments (or treatment sequence in the case of a study with a crossover design) such that each subject has an equal nonzero chance of being allocated to any given treatment (or treatment sequence) in the study. We may say, for example, that the first subject was randomized to Treatment A. If there are two treatments and a patient's chances of being assigned to each treatment are the same, we can randomize a patient using the flip of a fair coin. In such a case, the second subject could potentially also be randomized to Treatment A, but in the case of many entries we would see a balance in those randomized to A and B. *Clinical equipoise* (Freedman 1987), which means that there is genuine uncertainty in the expert medical community over whether a test treatment will be beneficial compared to the control, provides the ethical basis for equal randomization.

2.5.2 Why Randomization?

First, we need some background. The outcome of a study is the response that is measured (before and) after administration of a treatment; we expect it to be influenced differentially by the alternative treatments in the study. A prognostic factor is defined as a subject characteristic (such as sex) that may contribute to the outcome. Randomization avoids the potential for subjects with specific prognostic profiles to get assigned preferentially to a particular treatment (resulting in an "allocation bias"). Furthermore, and more importantly, the statistical methods that will be used to analyze the data are based on mathematical theories that assume that random allocation has occurred. If subjects were not randomly assigned to treatment, then such analyses would be less valid or invalid. Observational studies do not have randomization involved. Again, random allocation of treatments is ethical in clinical trials in the case of clinical equipoise—when the treating doctor does not know which of the treatments is best for the patients in terms of the ultimate benefits and risks (Doll 1998).

2.5.3 Logistics of Randomization and Blinding

Randomization of patients to treatment (or treatment sequence) avoids or minimizes *allocation bias*. A related but different method that often accompanies randomization is *blinding*. Blinding is a way to mask the treatment assignment and contains several layers. Basic blinding is implemented as subjects are recruited into the study, to avoid *selection bias*. During the randomization and study, we mask the subject, the investigator, or both to prevent them from knowing the (random) treatment assignment and avoid *assessment bias*. *Single-blind* trials are those where only subjects are masked. A *double-blind* trial refers to one where both subjects and investigators are masked. Some pharmaceutical companies also implement the so-called *triple-blinding* in which the project statistician is also masked when analyzing the data. In contrast, *open-label* trials are those where neither patients nor investigators are masked. Schultz et al. (1995) reanalyzed 250 randomized trials from 33 meta-analyses and found that treatment effects were 30%–40% larger in trials without adequate concealment of treatment allocation. Kunz and Oxman (1998) also reported empirical evidence of bias in trials without random allocation or adequate concealment of allocation.

2.5.3.1 The Process of Randomization

First, a person who is *not* involved in patient recruitment, the consent process, administrating treatment, or assessment of subjects creates a *randomization schedule*. This person is often the trial biostatistician. The randomization schedule is the sequential list of treatment assignments for subjects who will be enrolled in the study.

Randomization must involve an element of unpredictability. After the randomization schedule is created, the treatment allocation is fixed on the schedule. What is actually random (unpredictable) is the order in which subjects arrive for treatment. Therefore, it is important that the next treatment in sequence be kept confidential to avoid the possibility of *selection bias*. This fact should be communicated to the medical research staff and the patients.

Conventionally, the person who generated the randomization schedule also keeps the schedule (in a centralized location in the case of a multicenter trial). This person (or designee) is contacted once a subject is deemed eligible for the study and has provided consent. This person then informs the investigator or pharmacy of the subject's treatment assignment. Alternatively, sealed envelopes, vials, or medication bottles are numbered and kept by the investigator or pharmacy. These are then used successively as each eligible and consenting patient begins on the study. A sealed sequentially numbered envelope, for example, helps assure the confidentiality of the next randomization.

Many trials sponsored by the pharmaceutical industry now commonly use a centralized, automated, interactive voice or web response system (IVRS or IWRS) instead of a contact person. The IVRS or IWRS usually also provides 24-hour code-breaking capability for investigators when an emergency occurs. In a recent paper, Goodale and McEntegart (2013) described various sources of bias and how technology can be used to eliminate or reduce the risk of occurrence of bias. This paper also cited various references covering examples and the effects of bias. For example, Zhao, Hill, and Palesch (2012) used the Captopril Prevention Project trial as an example to describe how selection bias can occur when technology is not used for the implementation of randomization.

In summary, as presented in the study by Armitage (1982), randomization (i) helps to align treatment groups with similar distributions of prognostic factors; (ii) permits the use of probability theory to express quantitatively the extent to which any difference in response between treatment groups is likely to be due to chance; and (iii) allows various devices for masking the identity of treatment, including the possible use of a placebo, which are often essential for an unbiased assessment of efficacy by the subject or the observer, or both.

2.6 Methods for Randomization

We now turn our attention to several randomization methods and their merits, from simple to more sophisticated approaches. More detail on this topic can be found in Rosenberger and Lachin (2002). For any randomization method, we desire not only to achieve a certain fixed ratio of subjects in each treatment group but also to ensure that subject groups are similar with respect to prognostic factors such as age, stage or severity of disease, and many others.

2.6.1 Completely Randomized Design

For a randomized trial with two treatments with even allocation, the simplest method is to toss a fair (balanced) coin over and over again (for more than two groups, to roll a die). Although reasonable, these manual methods are rather antiquated. Computer generated random numbers are now commonly used instead. Completely randomized design, also called simple (unrestricted) randomization, is the design where no blocking or stratification is involved. The advantage of such a simple design is that each treatment assignment is completely unpredictable, hence with minimal chance of selection bias by investigators. For a large trial, the number of subjects in each treatment group will not be drastically different. However, for a trial with a small size or for an (early) interim analysis, the possibility exists that treatment groups will end up with considerably unequal numbers of subjects. For example, for a trial with 20 patients, the probability of getting 12 or more patients (60% or more) on a single treatment is approximately 50%. For a trial with 40 patients, the probability of getting 24 or more patients (60%) or more on a single treatment is approximately 27%. Additionally, sometimes known prognostic factors can be unevenly distributed in small groups, and a simple randomization may not distribute such factors evenly. In other words, without proper stratification, treatment groups also might be imbalanced with respect to influential prognostic factors. Therefore, blocked randomization and stratified randomization, or both combined, are often implemented in clinical trials (Homework 2.2).

2.6.2 Blocked Randomization

Blocked randomization is used to perform simple randomization within blocks in order to avoid severely imbalanced allocation to treatment groups. Suppose we have J treatments and s replicates. For a block size of s × J, we then produce a different simple randomization for each s × J patients. We should keep the block size confidential and especially not write it in the protocol. The block size should not be too small (e.g., s = 1 is not a good idea), nor should it be too large (e.g., s > 5 would be considered large). A small s makes the randomization sequence somewhat predictable. A large s, on the other hand, defeats the purpose of using blocks for balanced allocation. We also can vary s from block to block, which will then create a "varying block size randomization" design. Varying block size randomization, together with masking or blinding for double-blind trials, makes prediction of future allocations difficult, thus minimizing selection bias and achieving the desirable ratio of patient numbers between treatment groups (Homework 2.3).

2.6.3 Stratified Randomization

In clinical trials, we prefer to have similar treatment groups with regard to certain baseline characteristics of subjects. For example, in many instances gender and age relate to disease severity and outcome. If we recognize a factor that is known to influence the subject's outcome, it would be problematic if the treatment groups were not comparable in that prognostic factor. Even though there do exist methods of statistical analysis that can be used to address this issue, we would see a loss of statistical efficiency and would need to make additional efforts to convince others that the conclusion is valid. When such factors are chosen, strata are formed. Stratified randomization can be a complete (simple) randomization within each stratum. The randomization can also be a "blocked" (as in a group) randomization within each stratum, called "permuted blocks" by Armitage (1982). However, most believe it advisable to limit the number of strata in a feasible manner. This technique also critically relates to the overall number of subjects to be enrolled in the trial. For example, for a cancer trial that considers age (<55 vs. ≥55), gender (male vs. female), performance status (score 1–2 vs. 3–4), time since diagnosis (<6 months vs. ≥6 months), there will be $2 \times 2 \times 2 \times 2 = 16$ combinations for strata, each requiring a separate randomization. For many prognostic factors, we may consider another method for allocation of patients to treatment groups: the *minimization method*.

Aside: Stratified randomization in clinical trials is similar to the so-called randomized block design in classical experimental design, such as was used in agriculture, the agricultural "blocks" being analogous to the clinical strata, rather than to the blocks that are permutated for balanced allocation. The agricultural blocks are a fixed size, whereas the strata in clinical trials are initially of unknown size; the balancing therefore should occur in a sequential manner.

2.7 Minimization

When there are many prognostic factors to consider, often the need is to balance the marginal distributions rather than the joint distribution. That is, we desire to balance each of the factors individually and simultaneously, when the number of combinations of factors is too large to be feasible. The method of minimization works toward this goal.

The minimization method was first described by Taves (1974), then by Pocock and Simon (1975). This method may be viewed as a special form of adaptive design that is nonresponse dependent. (An example of response-dependent adaptive design is given in Appendix 3A.1 in Chapter 3. More about adaptive designs is discussed in later chapters with sequential designs and methods.) Patients are assigned to treatment as they are enrolled in the study, rather than through a preset randomization schedule. Treatment groups are balanced only with respect to the potential main effects of the prognostic factors. There is no need to prespecify the number of patients within each strata of each variable. We describe the method by a common case as follows.

Suppose we have two treatment groups, A and B, in a trial. Consider three prognostic factors that have I, J, and K levels (e.g., $I = J = K = 2$). At any time during the trial, let n_{ijk}^A represent the number of subjects randomized to Treatment A at levels i, j, and k of the prognostic factors, respectively, and n_{ijk}^B represent those within the same strata randomized to Treatment B, with $n_{ijk} = n_{ijk}^A + n_{ijk}^B$. Under simple stratification, we have $n_{ijk}^A \approx n_{ijk}^B$.

The notation n_{i++}^A represents the number of individuals at the ith level of the first prognostic factor that are randomized to Treatment A, summed over the second and third prognostic factors. The same is true for n_{i++}^B. These are the marginal totals for the first prognostic factor at level i in treatment groups A and B, respectively. To balance the marginal distribution of the first prognostic factor in treatment groups A and B is to ensure that $n_{i++}^A \approx n_{i++}^B$ for all i.

Likewise, to balance the second factor, we need to ensure $n_{+j+}^A \approx n_{+j+}^B$ for all j, and for the third factor, we need to reach $n_{++k}^A \approx n_{++k}^B$ for all k.

For each patient enrolled, we note their levels of the prognostic factors, say, i^*, j^*, and k^*, respectively. Calculate the quantity

$$G = \left(n_{i^*++}^A - n_{i^*++}^B\right) + \left(n_{+j^*+}^A - n_{+j^*+}^B\right) + \left(n_{++k^*}^A - n_{++k^*}^B\right) \tag{2.5}$$

G represents the total amount of imbalance. Treatment assignment depends on whether G is negative, positive, or zero. If G is negative, indicating a deficit of assignment to A, then the new patient is allocated to A (with probability p). If G is positive, meaning a deficit of assignment to B, then the patient is allocated to B (with probability p). If G equals zero, the treatment assignments are at equilibrium, and the patient is allocated to A or B (with initialization probability 1/2). Note that for the first patient the above quantity is zero. The probability $p = 2/3$ or $3/4$ might be a suitable choice to prevent advanced predictions of the next treatment assignment. Often, in practice, $p = 1$ when there is no such concern. However, the International Conference on Harmonisation (ICH) *E9, Statistical Principles for Clinical Trials*, recommends that a random element should be incorporated into deterministic dynamic allocation procedures like minimization (Lewis 1999).

The above method can easily accommodate many numbers of prognostic factors as well as different numbers of levels of each prognostic factor. Additionally, if balance is more important among some prognostic factors than others, the quantity above can be modified to be a weighted sum. The minimization method with a random element is commonly and most efficiently implemented by an automated IVRS/IWRS.

We now give an example for illustration. Suppose a trial with two treatment groups (experimental and control) has already enrolled 18 participants. Table 2.1 summarizes the three characteristics (sex, age range, and disease stage) for the 18 participants that the trial wishes to balance between treatment groups. If the next (19th) subject is male, aged 46, and at a moderate disease stage, the decision to allocate to the experimental or control group can be made by computing the imbalance quantity G (2.5) as illustrated below the table. In this case, G = –1, hence the 19th participant would be assigned to the experimental group.

As we can see from the illustration, if the weight to disease stage is double or more than that of age and sex as prognostic factors, the allocation could be different. This method can be generalized to more treatments. Other more complicated minimization methods also exist (see Cook and DeMets, 2007). A good review and recommendation can be found in Scott et al. (2002).

Note that minimization is a deterministic method in that the allocation of the next subject to treatment is determined by the previous allocations of subjects enrolled. Technically correct statistical analysis following minimization is complicated and involves simulation of multiple data sets (100,000) under the assumption of no treatment effect and the practiced allocation strategy. Then, observed results are compared to the distribution of simulated possible results in order to obtain a p-value. In practice, though, analyses may be conducted with the minimization factors used as covariates

TABLE 2.1

Example to Illustrate the Minimization Method

Prognostic Factor	Experimental Group	Control Group
Sex		
Male	4	5
Female	5	4
Age Range		
18–40	4	3
41–65	2	3
>65	3	3
Disease Stage		
Moderate	5	4
Severe	4	5

Note: If the 19th patient is male, aged 46, with moderate disease stage: Imbalance quantity = $(4 - 5) + (2 - 3) + (5 - 4) = -1$. Therefore, allocate the 19th patient to the experimental group.

in the model. Simulation studies have shown the power and type I error rate to be similar between these two approaches (e.g., Forsythe and Stitt 1977, Green et al. 2001). Senn (1995) even argued that factors used in the minimization must also be included in the analysis and that using minimization but not including the covariates in the model is not legitimate.

Concerns were raised (e.g., Berger 2006, 2011) that randomization with more restrictions such as blocked randomization and deterministic methods such as minimization without a random element preclude allocation concealment and invite selection bias by a sophisticated person who can figure out future treatment assignment when the trial is not masked. To alleviate such concerns, trials should be adequately designed and executed to mask the treatment assignment. Recent advances in technology, as described by Goodale and McEntegart (2013), should be utilized to achieve this goal. Setting the probability $p = 2/3$ or $4/5$ in the allocation of treatment (see the paragraph following Equation 2.5) is one way to incorporate a random element in the deterministic dynamic allocation procedure (Homework 2.4).

2.8 Table of Patient Demographics and Baseline Characteristics

The first table in the results section of a clinical trial paper often has a heading such as "Patient Demographics and Baseline Characteristics," and the display is often by treatment groups as well as with treatment groups combined. Sometimes the table also provides p-values for these baseline variables (covariates). In a clinical, nonrandomized study, showing p-values for comparability between groups is meaningful and very necessary to investigate possible *confounding factors*. However, if the trial is randomized (at least titled as such), then we should ask whether these p-values are meaningful. What is the intended purpose of such a table? Take a minute to contemplate this.

Such a table display may serve multiple purposes. The overall column obviously describes the enrolled participants so as to inform the reader about the applicability of the trial result to the medical practice in general (see Section 2.1, "External Validity"). The display by treatment groups, however, can be more interesting, especially when significance tests are performed for each baseline variable. Many authors have discussed this topic (e.g., Altman 1985, Senn 1989, and Begg 1990). One school of thought states that it is not meaningful to calculate p-values there, because we know the trial is randomized, and the characteristics are baseline values (without treatment effect), so the null hypothesis of no difference between groups is true. Therefore, any statistical significance indicated by a low p-value is simply a type I error, and it is thus pointless and should be avoided. Furthermore, if we examine many baseline variables, as this kind of table often does, we expect to find some "significance" by chance alone. For example, in the report of the Coronary Drug Project (1973), 420 drug-placebo comparisons on baseline characteristics were carried out. The authors correctly pointed out that they would "expect to find about 21 of the differences to be significant at the 0.05 level." They actually observed 22, and concluded that "... there is no evidence of lack of comparability of the treatment groups at baseline." Is this a correct conclusion? (The answer is no, as we explain in the next paragraph.)

Others may ask the question: How do we know the randomization process, as described, was actually carried out properly and that it worked as intended? The editor, the reader, and the FDA authority may wish to check on this by such a table display. In other words, the significance tests are meaningful for the hypothesis that the treatments are randomly allocated, or whether the supposedly randomized trial was in actuality a randomized trial. For the Coronary Drug Project mentioned above, the significance tests only indicated that the randomization was fair. Incidentally, more powerful approaches to analyzing these observed p-values for testing the null hypothesis of randomization also exist; for example, Schweder and Spjotvoll (1982) focused on this in greater detail.

However, if the purpose of doing significance tests here is to check randomization, then we can simply ask the patient irrelevant questions and test the distributions of answers to questions such as "What is your favorite color (or sport)?"—which carry no prognostic importance whatsoever to the outcome of the study. Obviously, the intention of the table is to examine the "baseline comparability," not merely for checking the fairness of randomization. What then, does a p-value tell us about a treatment group's comparability? Can we judge what factor to adjust in the statistical analysis by looking at the p-values? The answer to both questions is obviously no.

Baseline comparability of treatment groups may be represented by the treatment-covariate association. The p-values in the baseline table of a medical paper could not measure the strength of the treatment-covariate association; each p-value is simply testing the hypothesis of null association. If significance tests are not appropriate for assessing baseline comparability in RCTs, how should it be done? Altman (1985) recommended it be initially judged "using a combination of clinical knowledge and common sense." Here, previous experience plays a key role. The actual implication of comparability or lack thereof is whether to adjust for a covariate or not in the analysis.

In a (truly) randomized trial, we can choose to analyze the treatment effect without any covariate and the conclusions will be valid, irrespective of the observed treatment-covariate association. In this regard, the p-values in the baseline table of a medical paper are not needed. However, the observed p-value for the treatment-covariate association is very informative about the probability, say, that a significant treatment effect is a false positive. For example, suppose that in a trial, the treatment effect is on the borderline of being significant, and that the treatments are not well distributed with respect to some covariate that is strongly prognostic to the outcome. Then conditional on the observed treatment-covariate distribution, the probability of a significant treatment effect under the null hypothesis will be much higher than the nominal significance level. The converse is true when the treatments are especially well balanced with respect to the covariate (Begg 1990).

As a common practice, we usually adjust a prognostic factor that is unbalanced between the groups. In Chapter 5, we write an analysis of covariance (ANCOVA) model to demonstrate the appropriateness of the above practice. We show that the degree of adjustment and the variance reduction depends on two factors: the covariate's correlation or association with the outcome variable and the between-group imbalance. The p-values in the baseline table of a medical paper have no bearing on the adjustment of covariates.

Homework 2.1

Write out the formula in Equation 2.4 for a control group labeled as Y. Discuss how randomization in treatment allocation and blinding in assessing treatment effects can help cancel out the bias of the effect of regression to the mean.

Homework 2.2

1. Use the SAS® or R software to generate a completely randomized allocation schedule for a trial with total sample size N = 50, two treatment groups, and even allocation design. Comment on the actual sample size of each group.

   Hint: Use the R software to generate a list of 50 random numbers from the uniform (0,1) distribution. Assign Patient 1 the first random number, Patient 2 the second random number, etc. If a patient's random number is <0.5, then assign that patient to Treatment A; otherwise, assign the patient to Treatment B. SAS has a procedure called PROC PLAN that you may also use.

2. Use either a mathematical derivation or run your computer program repeatedly 10,000 times to show that in this case (N = 50) the probability is greater than 5% that the design will end up as an uneven treatment allocation in the ratio of 18:32 or more extreme.

Homework 2.3

Use the SAS or R software to generate a blocked randomization schedule for a trial with total sample size N = 180, three treatment groups, and an even allocation design. Vary the block size by permuting s = 1, 2, 3. How many blocks will there be? Comment on the actual sample size of each group.

Homework 2.4*

Suppose that 32 patients will be recruited for a clinical trial comparing Treatments A and B. After completing the consent process for these patients, they will be allocated to one of the treatments. Suppose that age (categories 18–25, 26–39, 40–60) and gender (M, F) are expected to be important prognostic factors for the outcome being studied. Using the minimization approach, create a randomization schedule using an initialization probability of 1/2 and the probability of 1 afterwards. Use the following uniform random numbers in the allocation procedure (rather than generating your own):

0.26, 0.69, 0.11, 0.51, 0.22, 0.56, 0.23, 0.98, 0.11, 0.43, 0.53, 0.98, 0.29 and 0.23

Note: You should not need to do any computer programming for this problem.

The following are the ages and genders of the 32 subjects in the order in which they were enrolled in the study:

ID	Age	Gender
1	26	F
2	32	F
3	18	M
4	29	F
5	35	F
6	35	M
7	38	F
8	55	M
9	56	M
10	34	F
11	22	M

Continued

---

* Homework 2.4 was contributed by Pamela Ohman-Strickland.

ID	Age	Gender
12	22	F
13	23	F
14	35	F
15	34	F
16	22	F
17	34	M
18	56	F
19	59	F
20	29	M
21	45	F
22	43	F
23	33	F
24	23	M
25	49	F
26	51	F
27	23	F
28	38	F
29	34	M
30	19	F
31	39	F
32	40	M

According to the randomization schedule you created:

1. How many subjects are allocated to Treatments A and B within each age-gender subcategory?
2. How many subjects are allocated to Treatments A and B within each age group?
3. How many within each gender group?
4. How many overall?

References

Adami S, Passeri M, Ortolani S, Broggini M, Carratelli L, Caruso I, and Gandolini G. (1995). Effects of oral alendronate and intranasal salmon calcitonin on bone mass and biochemical markers of bone turnover in postmenopausal women with osteoporosis. *Bone* 17: 383–390.

Altman DG. (1985). Comparability of randomized groups. *The Statistician* 34: 125–136.

Armitage P. (1982). The role of randomization in clinical trials. *Statistics in Medicine* 1: 345–352.

Bland JM and Altman DG. (1994). Regression towards the mean. *British Medical Journal* 308: 1499.

Begg CB. (1990). Significance tests of covariate imbalance in clinical trials. *Controlled Clinical Trials* 11: 223–225.

Berger VW. (2006). Misguided precedent is not a reason to use permuted blocks. *Headache* 46: 1210–1212.

Berger VW. (2011). Minimization: not all it's cracked up to be. *Clinical Trials* 8: 443.

Cook TD and DeMets DL. (2007). *Introduction to Statistical Methods for Clinical Trials*. New York: Chapman & Hall/CRC.

Cummings SR, Palermo L, Browner W, Marcus R, Wallace R, Pearson J, and Blackwell T. (2000). Monitoring osteoporosis therapy with bone mineral density: misleading changes and regression to the mean. *Journal of the American Medical Association* 283: 1318–1321.

Daniel WW. (2009). *Biostatistics: A Foundation for Analysis in the Health Sciences*. New York: Wiley.

Doll R. (1998). Controlled trials: the 1948 watershed. *British Medical Journal* 317: 1217–1220.

Downs JR, and Clearfield M. (1998). Primary prevention of acute coronary events with lovastatin in men and women with average cholesterol levels: results of AFCAPS/TexCAPS. Air Force/Texas Coronary Atherosclerosis Prevention Study. *Journal of the American Medical Association* 27: 1615–1622.

Evidence-Based Medicine Working Group. (1992). Evidence-based medicine – a new approach to teaching the practice of medicine. *Journal of the American Medical Association* 268: 2420–2425.

Featherstone K and Donovan JL. (1998). Random allocation or allocation at random? Patients' perspective of participation in randomized controlled trial. *British Medical Journal* 317: 1177–1180.

Friedman LM, Furberg CD, and DeMets DL. (1996). *Fundamentals of Clinical Trials*. New York: Springer.

Forsythe AB and Stitt FW. (1977). *Randomization or Minimization in the Treatment Assignment of Patient Trials: Validity and Power of Tests. Technical Report No. 28.* Health Sciences Computing Facility, Los Angeles: UCLA.

Freedman, B (1987). Equipoise and the ethics of clinical research. *The New England Journal of Medicine*, 317: 141–145.

Goodale H and McEntegart D. (2013). The role of technology in avoiding bias in the design and execution of clinical trials. *Open Access Journal of Clinical Trials* 5: 13–21. http://dx.doi.org/10.2147/OAJCT.S40760.

Green H, McEntegart DJ, Byrom B, Ghani S, and Shepherd S. (2001). Minimization in crossover trials with non-prognostic strata: theory and practical application. *Journal of Clinical Pharmacy and Therapeutics* 26: 121–128.

Horton R. (2000). Common sense and figures: the rhetoric of validity in medicine (Bradford Hill Memorial Lecture 1999). *Statistics in Medicine* 19: 3149–3164.

Julian DG and Pocock SJ. (1997). Interpreting a trial report. In *Clinical Trials in Cardiology*. Pitt B, Julian D, and Pocock S (eds.). London: WB Saunders.

Kunz R and Oxman AD. (1998). The unpredictability paradox: review of empirical comparisons of randomised and non-randomised clinical trials. *British Medical Journal* 317: 1185–1190.

Lewis JA. (1999). Statistical principles for clinical trials (ICH E9): an introductory note on an international guideline. *Statistics in Medicine* 18: 1903–1942.

Pocock SJ and Simon R. (1975). Sequential treatment assignment with balancing for prognostic factors in the controlled clinical trial. *Biometrics* 31: 103–115.

Rosenberger W and Lachin JM. (2002). *Randomization in Clinical Trials: Theory and Practice*. New York: John Wiley and Sons.

Rothwell PM. (2005). External validity of randomized controlled trials: "To whom do the results of this trial apply?" *Lancet* 365: 82–93.

Schultz KF, Chalmers I, Hayes RJ, and Altman DG. (1995). Empirical evidence of bias. Dimensions of methodological quality associated with estimates of treatment effects in controlled trials. *Journal of the American Medical Association* 273: 408–412.

Schweder T and Spjotvoll E. (1982). Plots of *P*-values to evaluate many tests simultaneously. *Biometrika* 69: 493–502.

Scott NW, McPherson CG, Ramsay CR, and Campbell MK. (2002). The method of minimization for allocation to clinical trials: a review. *Controlled Clinical Trials* 23: 662–674.

Senn SJ. (1989). Covariate imbalance and random allocation in clinical trials. *Statistics in Medicine* 8: 467–475.

Senn SJ. (1995). A personal view of some controversies in allocating treatment to patients in clinical trials. *Statistics in Medicine* 14: 2661–2674.

Simvastatin Scandinavian Survival Study Group. (1994). Randomised trial of cholesterol lowering in 4444 patients with coronary heart disease: the Scandinavian Simvastatin Survival Study (4S). *Lancet* 19; 344: 1383–1389.

Taves DR. (1974). Minimization: a new method of assigning patients to treatment and control groups. *Clinical Pharmacology and Therapeutics* 15: 443–453.

The Coronary Drug Project Research Group. (1973). The coronary drug project: design, methods and baseline results. *Circulation* 47 & 48 (Suppl. 1): I-1–I-50.

Zhao W, Hill MD, and Palesch Y. (2012). Minimal sufficient balance – a new strategy to balance baseline covariates and preserve randomness of treatment allocation. *Statistical Methods in Medical Research* January 26, 2012.

3

Efficiency with Trade-Offs and Crossover Designs

The two primary concerns of statistical design are *bias* and *efficiency*. We have discussed the concept of bias and methods to help avoid or minimize bias in the last chapter. In this chapter, we explore the concept of efficiency. We begin with two simple examples. In each example, we see that sample size and variance of the outcome variable (endpoint) play the main roles in defining statistical efficiency. Efficiency gains also involve trade-offs when considering trial design. We use the crossover design for an illustration of the trade-offs in efficiency. The crossover design is also useful as a way to introduce the analysis of variance (ANOVA) cell-means model. In Appendices 3.1 through 3.3, we briefly introduce designs that maximize benefit of treatment, for example measuring by the expected number of responders, as an alternative to efficiency for the purpose of designing trials optimally.

3.1 Statistical Efficiency of a Design

We first consider two conceptual examples:

Example 3.1

Consider a study to compare two treatments, X and Y. Let the endpoint be a continuous variable so that the mean difference is the parameter of interest. We have two design options: For Design A, we recruit n pairs of identical twins and randomly assign each sibling to a treatment group. (If one sibling gets treatment X randomly, the other will automatically get treatment Y.) For Design B, we randomize 2n unrelated individuals with 1:1 (equal) allocation to the treatment groups, with the same eligibility as in Design A. Assume both designs use the same bias-avoiding procedures. Which design is more efficient?

Given that Design A uses twins, each member of the pair serves as the control for the other member of the pair, whereas in Design B the 2n individuals are unrelated. Design A will use a paired t-test, and

Design B will use a two-sample t-test to compare the means. The paired t-test statistic is larger than its two-sample t-test statistic counterpart because, although the two statistics have the same numerator (sample mean difference), the paired t-test has a smaller denominator (standard error). Design A is thus more efficient (Homework 3.1).

However, the smaller standard error (higher efficiency) resulting from correlation between the twins comes with a trade-off: paired twins are more difficult to recruit than unrelated individuals.

Example 3.2

Consider a randomized study to compare two treatment groups, again with a continuous outcome variable. Let the total sample size be fixed and, for simplicity, be large enough that we can comfortably use the standardized normal distribution z-test (rather than a t-test). We have two design options. Design A uses 1:1 allocation and Design B uses 1:2 (unequal) allocation. Assume the outcome variable has the same variance in both treatment groups. Which design is more efficient?

Design A is more efficient because a statistical test with a balanced design has a smaller variance. The proof is shown in Appendix 3.1.

Discussion: Sometimes we would like to place more patients in the group receiving the investigational medicine than in the control (e.g., placebo) to gain more knowledge about the new compound. In that case, we may use a less efficient unequal allocation. Also note that an unequal allocation design is more efficient when the variances are not the same in the treatment groups. In this case, more patients are needed for the treatment group with greater variance. See Appendix 3.2 for details.

Let the treatment effect be estimated by the observed $\hat{\delta}$ and its *standard error* (se) be expressed as $\mathrm{se}(\hat{\delta})$. From the above examples involving t-tests and the z-test, and in general, the form of a Wald test or a score test is

$$T = \frac{\hat{\delta}}{\mathrm{s.e.}(\hat{\delta})}$$

We see that T increases as $\mathrm{s.e.}(\hat{\delta})$ decreases, implying a more significant result. This would then imply a higher power. The above se usually involves sample size n and an estimate of the population standard deviation (SD). Aiming for a target statistical power, a more efficient design means fewer patients are needed. Alternatively, with a fixed sample size, a more efficient design provides the study with a greater power. In Chapter 4, we discuss the topic of sample size and power. Before we proceed, we look at the cross-over design. This design provides good illustrations for (i) another kind of randomization—randomizing the treatment sequence, (ii) the commonly used concept of the ANOVA cell-means model, and (iii) some trade-offs to be considered in a trial design to gain efficiency.

3.2 Crossover Designs

Crossover designs are commonly used in Phase I *bioavailability* (BA) and *bioequivalence* (BE) pharmacology trials to study the pharmacokinetics (PK)—absorption, metabolism, distribution, and elimination (AMDE)—of a new compound in the human body. PK variables of interest include the measurements of peak concentration in blood or urine, time to peak concentration, half-life, and exposure (area under the curve, or AUC) within a certain period of time, usually 24 or 48 hours. A characteristic of a crossover design is that each patient receives the test compound as well as the control agent. In this way, each patient serves as the control for himself or herself. There are many varieties; we study the simplest 2 × 2 crossover for the purpose of highlighting the trade-offs with efficiency (Table 3.1).

For example, if $n_1 = n_2 = n = 10$, then a total of 20 subjects are in the trial, where all 20 receive A and also B. (In contrast, for a parallel group design with 20 subjects per treatment group, there would be 40 subjects in total.) Subjects are randomized into the two sequences (AB or BA). The major advantage is an increase in efficiency (i.e., a decrease in number of subjects). This is due to *pairing*, as we saw in Section 3.1 when we compared the paired t-test to the independent t-test. A trade-off here is the increase in study duration—two periods, plus a *washout period* in between. In addition, a major concern of a crossover design is that, if the washout period is not sufficiently long, based on the half-life of the compounds under study, there may be a *residual effect* from the treatment in the first period added to the (direct) treatment effect of the second period. (For a 3 × 3 crossover, there would be first-order and second-order residual effects to be concerned about.) Moreover, the residual treatment effects, if they exist, may not be equal in magnitude for the two treatment sequences. Even if there is no residual effect, the experimenter should also check whether a confounding *period effect* is a possibility (e.g., temporal or seasonal effects if the periods occur over different times). Statistically, one can test whether the period effect is (statistically) significant or not. But we should note that this test may not have adequate power to test the issue. The statistical nonsignificance does not prove nonexistence of an effect.

TABLE 3.1

A 2 × 2 Crossover Layout

Sequence	Patient	Period 1 Washout Period	Period 2
1	1	A	B
1	2	A	B
1	n_1	A	B
2	1	B	A
2	2	B	A
2	n_2	B	A

Note. Usually, $n_1 = n_2 = n$ (balanced allocation is usually most efficient).

Note that in the literature *residual effect* and *carryover effect* are used interchangeably, and treatment *sequence* and *group* are also used interchangeably in this context.

After the washout period, and before receiving the second period treatment, subjects' condition should return to the same baseline as in the first period. This is the main reason why the crossover design is suitable for BA/BE studies with healthy volunteers, where returning to the baseline condition after a period of time is achievable. However, this may be greatly influenced by the pharmacokinetics (how long the agent lasts) and the pharmacodynamics (how long the biological effects of the agent last). For example, a cytotoxic agent may clear quickly, whereas the biological effect may last weeks. It is obvious that crossover design is never used in survival studies. Drugs that elicit an immune response are also not ideal for crossover designs. More discussion on this topic, including drawbacks and limitations of crossover designs, can be found in Louis et al. (1984).

3.3 Analysis of 2 × 2 Crossover Designs

First, consider a model for a general crossover design. Let y_{ijk} be the continuous outcome of the subject k in treatment sequence/group i and period j. A linear model for a general crossover design is expressed in the following

$$y_{ijk} = E(y_{ijk}) + e_{ijk}$$

where

$$E(y_{ijk}) = \mu + \pi_j + \tau_{d[i,j]} + \lambda_{d[i, j-1]} \tag{3.1}$$

and e_{ijk} is the random error with normal distribution $N(0, \sigma^2)$, μ is the grand mean, π_j is the j th *period effect*, $\tau_{d[i,j]}$ is the *(direct) treatment effect* from sequence i and period j, and $\lambda_{d[i, j-1]}$ is the *residual effect* from the previous period on the same subject. Note that, if there is no residual effect ($\lambda_{d[i, j-1]} = 0$) and no period effect ($\pi_j = 0$), then the above model reduces to a one-way ANOVA with a paired-data design.

For a 2 × 2 crossover design, $i = j = 2$. The analysis can be conveniently carried out by a series of t-tests (or rank tests when the distribution is skewed), with the expansion of the above expression to the following cell-means model. That is, in each (Group, Period) cell, we write down the mean of the observations, as follows:

Sequence	Period 1	Period 2	
1 (AB)	$\mu + \pi_1 + \tau_1$	$\mu + \pi_2 + \tau_2 + \lambda_1$	
2 (AB)	$\mu + \pi_1 + \tau_2$	$\mu + \pi_2 + \tau_1 + \lambda_2$	(3.2)

The first step is to test for the equality of residual (carryover) effects: $\lambda_1 = \lambda_2$. (Note that this is a weaker condition than no residual effects, $\lambda_1 = \lambda_2 = 0$.) This test can be done as follows. We sum the measurements over the two periods for each subject of the two treatment sequences:

$$t_{1k} = y_{11k} + y_{12k}$$

$$t_{2k} = y_{21k} + y_{22k}$$

(3.3)

Note that

$$E(t_{1k}) = 2\mu + \pi_1 + \pi_2 + \tau_1 + \tau_2 + \lambda_1$$

$$E(t_{2k}) = 2\mu + \pi_1 + \pi_2 + \tau_1 + \tau_2 + \lambda_2$$

Hence, $E(t_{1k} - t_{2k}) = \lambda_1 - \lambda_2$. We can compare the sums t_{1k} and t_{2k} by an independent t-test and obtain T_λ with $n_1 + n_2 - 2$ degrees of freedom (df). Grizzle (1965) suggested to perform this preliminary test at the two-sided $\alpha = 0.10$ level.

The second step is to test for the equality of treatment effects: $\tau_1 = \tau_2$, assuming *equal* residual effects $\lambda_1 = \lambda_2$ (tested by the previous step).

We subtract the measurements between the two periods for each subject of the two treatment sequences:

$$d_{1k} = y_{11k} - y_{12k}$$

$$d_{2k} = y_{21k} - y_{22k}$$

(3.4)

We find:

$$E(d_{1k}) = \pi_1 - \pi_2 + \tau_1 - \tau_2 - \lambda_1$$

$$E(d_{2k}) = \pi_1 - \pi_2 - \tau_1 + \tau_2 - \lambda_2$$

Therefore, $E(d_{1k} - d_{2k}) = 2(\tau_1 - \tau_2)$, since $\lambda_1 = \lambda_2$. We can compare the differences d_{1k} and d_{2k} by an independent t-test and obtain T_τ with $df = n_1 + n_2 - 2$. If the residual effects are not equal, then $E(d_{1k} - d_{2k}) = 2(\tau_1 - \tau_2) - (\lambda_1 - \lambda_2) = (2\tau_1 + \lambda_2) - (2\tau_2 + \lambda_1)$. In this case, the residual effects are *confounded* with the direct treatment effects; hence, we cannot separate τ_1 and λ_2, τ_2 and λ_1.

We can further test the equality of the period effect $\pi_1 = \pi_2$, assuming *no* residual effects $\lambda_1 = \lambda_2 = 0$. To do this, we only need to reverse the second difference in (3.4). Let

$$c_{1k} = d_{1k} = y_{11k} - y_{12k}$$

$$c_{2k} = -d_{2k} = y_{22k} - y_{21k}$$

(3.5)

We find $E(c_{1k} - c_{2k}) = 2(\pi_1 - \pi_2)$. Therefore, we can compare the differences c_{1k} and c_{2k} by an independent t-test and obtain T_π with $df = n_1 + n_2 - 2$. (If the residual effects exist, then they are *confounded* with the period effect.)

TABLE 3.2

A 2 × 2 Crossover Trial of Acute Bronchial Asthma

	Sequence 1 (AB)				Sequence 2 (BA)			
Subject	Period 1	Period 2	Total	Difference	Subject	Period 1	Period 2	Total	Difference
1	1.28	1.33	2.61	−0.05	9	3.06	1.38	4.44	1.68
2	1.6	2.21	3.81	−0.61	10	2.68	2.1	4.78	0.58
3	2.46	2.43	4.89	0.03	11	2.6	2.32	4.92	0.28
4	1.41	1.81	3.22	−0.4	12	1.48	1.3	2.78	0.18
5	1.4	0.85	2.25	0.55	13	2.08	2.34	4.42	−0.26
6	1.12	1.2	2.32	−0.08	14	2.72	2.48	5.2	0.24
7	0.9	0.9	1.8	0	15	1.94	1.11	3.05	0.83
8	2.41	2.79	5.2	−0.38	16	3.35	3.23	6.58	0.12
					17	1.16	1.25	2.41	−0.09

Source: Jones, B., and Kenward, M. G., *Design and Analysis of Cross-Over Trials*, Chapman and Hall, New York, 1989.

Note: The outcome variable is the forced expired volume (liters) in one second (or FEV_1).

Example 3.3

In this example, we examine the data in Table 3.2. For this data set, $T_\lambda = -1.623$ with $n_1 + n_2 - 2 = 15$ *df* (p-value > 0.10). Thus, we proceed to test for equal direct treatment effects by $T_\tau = -2.162$ with 15 *df* (p < 0.05). Furthermore, we test the equality of the period effect $\pi_1 = \pi_2$, assuming *no* residual effects $\lambda_1 = \lambda_2 = 0$, by $T_\pi = 1.172$ with 15 *df* (p > 0.20) (Homework 3.2).

Appendix 3.1: Efficiency of the 1:1 Allocation Assuming Equal Variance

Compare the means of the primary endpoint of two independent treatment groups with a common variance. Show that a balanced design is more efficient than an imbalanced design. In particular, show that a 1:1 allocation is more efficient than a 1:2 allocation.

Proof:

Let $x_1, x_2, \ldots, x_{n1}$ be the n_1 samples from the treatment group X, and $y_1, y_2, \ldots, y_{n2}$ be the n_2 samples from the treatment group Y. $N = n_1 + n_2$. Assume X and Y are independent and normally distributed with means μ_x and μ_y, respectively, with common known variance σ^2. To test the hypothesis of $\mu_x = \mu_y$, the z-test statistic is

$$Z = \frac{\bar{X} - \bar{Y}}{\sqrt{\dfrac{\sigma^2}{n_1} + \dfrac{\sigma^2}{n_2}}} = \sqrt{\frac{n_1 n_2}{n_1 + n_2}} \frac{\bar{X} - \bar{Y}}{\sigma} \qquad (3A.1)$$

If $n_1 = n_2 = N/2$, then $\sqrt{\dfrac{n_1 n_2}{n_1 + n_2}} = \sqrt{\dfrac{N}{4}}$.

If $n_1 = N/3$, $n_2 = 2N/3$, then $\sqrt{\dfrac{n_1 n_2}{n_1 + n_2}} = \sqrt{\dfrac{2N}{9}}$.

Since $1/4 > 2/9$, then the 1:1 allocation results in a larger Z-statistic.

In general, let $n_1 = g \times N$, then $\dfrac{n_1 n_2}{n_1 + n_2} = \dfrac{g(1-g)N^2}{N} = g(1-g)N$.

Find the maximum of $g(1-g)$ by solving $\dfrac{dg(1-g)}{dg} = 0$, yielding $g = 1/2$. Therefore, $g = 1/2$ maximizes Z.

Appendix 3.2: Optimal Allocation under Unequal Variance

Using the above setting, let σ_X^2 and σ_Y^2 be the variances of the treatment groups X and Y, respectively. Suppose $\sigma_X^2 \neq \sigma_Y^2$ are known. The z-test statistic for the hypothesis of $\mu_x = \mu_y$ is

$$Z = \frac{\bar{X} - \bar{Y}}{\sqrt{\dfrac{\sigma_X^2}{n_1} + \dfrac{\sigma_Y^2}{n_2}}} \qquad (3A.2)$$

To achieve the maximum power, we would minimize $\dfrac{\sigma_X^2}{n_1} + \dfrac{\sigma_Y^2}{n_2}$ by choosing appropriate n_1 and n_2 subject to $n_1 + n_2 = N$, a prefixed constant. Show that the optimal allocation to treatment group X is $n_1 = g \times N$, where $g = \dfrac{\sigma_X}{\sigma_X + \sigma_Y}$. Equation 3A.1 is a special case where $\sigma_X = \sigma_Y$.

The proof is a homework assignment (Homework 3.3).

Appendix 3.3: Optimizing Number of Responders

The above discussion on optimal efficiency was designed to maximize the power of testing the hypothesis of equal means of the primary endpoint of two treatment groups by optimally allocating the sample sizes n_1 and n_2 to the two treatment groups, subject to $n_1 + n_2 = N$, a prefixed total N subjects. It boils down to minimizing the denominator of the Z-statistic in Equation 3A.2. There is also another kind of strategy that focuses on maximizing, not the power, but the expected number of "responders" for the trial, subject to a prefixed total N and fixed denominator of Z in Equation 3A.2. The rationale for this kind of strategy is based on optimizing ethics rather than optimizing efficiency. Below is an example from Biswas and Mandal (2004).

Suppose that a smaller value is more desirable to patients, and that there is a threshold constant c such that the subject is a responder if the endpoint value is less than c. The probability of a response in group X is $P(X<c) = \Phi\left(\dfrac{c-\mu_X}{\sigma_X}\right)$, where $\Phi(\cdot)$ is the cumulative density function (cdf) of the standard normal distribution. The same is true for group Y. We then maximize the total expected number of responders by choosing n_1 and n_2

$$\max\left\{n_1\,\Phi\left(\frac{c-\mu_X}{\sigma_X}\right) + n_2\,\Phi\left(\frac{c-\mu_X}{\sigma_Y}\right)\right\} \tag{3A.3}$$

subject to $n_1 + n_2 = N$, as well as $\dfrac{\sigma_X^2}{n_1} + \dfrac{\sigma_Y^2}{n_2} = K$. Both N and K are prefixed constants. The restriction on $\dfrac{\sigma_X^2}{n_1} + \dfrac{\sigma_Y^2}{n_2}$ will preserve a specified level of power for the test of equal means. The solution of Equation 3A.3 with the restrictions yields g, the optimal allocation proportion of subjects to treatment group X, as

$$g = \frac{\sigma_X\sqrt{\Phi\left(\dfrac{c-\mu_Y}{\sigma_Y}\right)}}{\sigma_X\sqrt{\Phi\left(\dfrac{c-\mu_Y}{\sigma_Y}\right)} + \sigma_Y\sqrt{\Phi\left(\dfrac{c-\mu_X}{\sigma_X}\right)}} \tag{3A.4}$$

Proof:
Homework 3.4.

In practice, the design is implemented by assuming some initial values, then estimating the parameters using the available data up to the first cohort of patients, and finally plugging them into Equation 3A.4 to find the optimal allocation proportion to treatment X for the next cohort of patients. Relating this procedure to the minimization method for sequential allocation of the next patient based on balancing the distribution of baseline covariates of previous enrollments (see Chapter 2), this procedure is a response-adaptive design for continuous endpoints. Other designs of this kind include Zelen's (1969) "play the winner rule."

Homework 3.1

Review the independent t-test and the paired t-test statistics and show the answer statement for Example 3.1.

TABLE 3.3

Weight Loss Data (kg)

	Sequence 1 (DP)				Sequence 2 (PD)			
Subject (k)	Period 1 (y_{11k})	Period 2 (y_{12k})	Total (t_{1k})	Difference (d_{1k})	Subject (k)	Period 1 (y_{21k})	Period 2 (y_{22k})	Total (t_{2k})	Difference (d_{2k})
1	1.1	0.0	1.1	1.1	6	−0.2	0.1	−0.1	−0.3
2	1.3	−0.3	1.0	1.6	7	0.6	0.5	1.1	0.1
3	1.0	0.6	1.6	0.4	8	0.9	1.6	2.5	−0.7
4	1.7	0.3	2.0	1.4	9	−2.0	−0.5	−2.5	−1.5
5	1.4	−0.7	0.7	2.1					

Homework 3.2[*]

Table 3.3 (Weight Loss Data) displays outcome data and calculations of Equations 3.3 and 3.4 from a clinical trial on weight loss (kg) with the test drug mCPP versus placebo using a 2 × 2 crossover design. The test drug mCPP is denoted by D (drug) and the placebo by P.

1. First, we simply assume that there are no carryover and no period effects. Because this is a small data set, we prefer to carry out the basic nonparametric sign test for equal treatment effects. Readers should review the sign test from an introductory level statistics textbook (Daniel 2009; see also Chapter 2) and apply it to this data.

2. Second, use the cell-means model to test the hypothesis regarding the assumption of equal carryover effect, whether there is a treatment effect, and whether there is a period effect (with necessary assumptions) by independent t-tests (or rank tests if you prefer, due to the small sample size).

Homework 3.3

Prove the assertion of Appendix 3.2.

---

[*] Homework problem 3.2 was contributed by Dirk F. Moore.

Homework 3.4

Prove the assertion of Appendix 3.3.

References

Biswas A and Mandal S. (2004). Optimal adaptive designs in Phase III clinical trials for continuous responses with covariates. In *m0Da 7—Advances in Model-Oriented Design and Analysis*, Di Bucchianico A, Lauter H, and Wynn HP (Eds.), Heidelberg, Germany: Physica-Verlag; 51–58.

Daniel WW. (2009). *Biostatistics: A Foundation for Analysis in the Health Sciences.* New York: Wiley.

Grizzle JE. (1965). The two-period change-over design and its use in clinical trials. *Biometrics* 21: 467–480.

Jones B and Kenward MG. (1989). *Design and Analysis of Cross-Over Trials.* New York: Chapman and Hall.

Louis TA, Lavori PW, Bailar JC, and Polansky M. (1984). Crossover and self-controlled designs in clinical research. *New England Journal of Medicine* 310: 24–31.

Zelen M. (1969). Play the winner rule and the controlled clinical trial. *Journal of the American Statistical Association* 64: 131–146.

4

Sample Size and Power Calculations

Some authors choose to refer to the topic of sample size calculation as sample size *estimation*. This word choice is understandable because the calculation of the sample size for a clinical trial is based on design parameters whose values are *estimated* from previous data, or some other form of external information or assumptions. On the other hand, some authors prefer to use the term *calculation* for sample size to distinguish from the estimation of a model parameter in the context of making statistical inferences; these estimated values are usually assumed as fixed in the calculation, and seldom considered for their uncertainty. We use calculation and estimation interchangeably in this book.

In previous chapters, we discussed how clinical trials should be designed to minimize potential bias and to balance efficiency and generalizability (homogeneous versus heterogeneous samples). We should also check feasibility and ensure enough resources are available to conduct the study, in order to detect a clinically meaningful treatment effect that impacts medical practice, which is the ultimate goal of a clinical trial. The aspects of feasibility and resources are also relevant to sample size and study power.

In Chapter 3, we briefly discussed the concept of efficiency of a trial in terms of sample size and power. If one design, say Design A, can achieve the same power to detect the same effect size as another design, say, Design B, but with a smaller sample size, then Design A is more efficient. Equivalently, if Design A, with the same sample size, can achieve a higher power than Design B can, then Design A is more efficient.

When the sample size is inadequate, the study is underpowered. An underpowered study will render inconclusive results, that is, the study may not be able to detect an existing important treatment effect. On the other hand, when the sample size is too large, the study is overpowered. An overpowered study wastes resources and affects its feasibility. That is, it may be unaffordable or not fundable or it may detect a small, nonmeaningful treatment effect. The question is: how can we design a trial with an appropriate sample size that is "just right?"

4.1 Fundamentals

Readers are expected to have understood the basics of hypothesis testing, including the notion of a null hypothesis (H_0) versus an alternative hypothesis (H_A), and the associated type I error (false positive) rate (often denoted as α) and type II error (false negative) rate (often denoted as β), and power (which equals $1 - \beta$). A two-sided test at an α level, or a one-sided test at an $\alpha/2$ level is commonly used in industrial and regulatory practice, but not necessarily followed by academic studies that are more exploratory in nature.

For the interplay of α and β, see www.intuitor.com/statistics/CurveApplet. html/. It gives a dynamic pictorial description and applet. Conventionally, α is set to be 1% or 5%, and β may be 10%, 15%, or 20%.

4.2 Comparing Means for Continuous Outcomes

For a randomized design with an equal allocation, which compares two parallel (independent) treatment groups with a continuous outcome, let $Y_{11}, \ldots, Y_{n1}$ be the n independent observations from Treatment 1 and $Y_{12}, \ldots, Y_{n2}$ be the other n independent observations from Treatment 2, so that the total sample size is N = 2n. Y could also be a change or percent change from baseline for each patient's laboratory or clinical measurements. We would like to test the null hypothesis of equal means as denoted by

$$H_0: \Delta = \mu_1 - \mu_2 = 0 \qquad (4.1)$$

The difference of the sample means $\hat{\Delta} = \bar{Y}_1 - \bar{Y}_2$ is the estimated treatment effect. We apply *large sample theory* to the sample means so that there is no need to assume the parent distribution is normal, but an equal variance for the distribution of the two groups ($= \sigma^2$) is a convenient assumption. Recall that this equal variance leads to the optimal balanced allocation $n_1 = n_2 = n$ (see Chapter 3). Let s^2 be the sample variance estimator pooled from both groups. The squared standard error (se) of $\hat{\Delta} = \bar{Y}_1 - \bar{Y}_2$ then is equal to $2s^2/n$ and the Wald test statistic is

$$T = \frac{\hat{\Delta}}{se(\hat{\Delta})} \qquad (4.2)$$

T follows the t distribution with $2(n - 1)$ degrees of freedom. With a large sample size, the t distribution approaches the normal distribution. When designing a study, we assume a known value for σ^2. Then T = Z (replacing s^2 in T with σ^2), whose distribution is the standard normal, N(0, 1), under the null hypothesis. As seen in Appendix 3.3 (in Chapter 3), its *cumulative distribution*

TABLE 4.1

Commonly Used Quantiles of the
Standard Normal Distribution

$z_{0.01}$	$=$	2.326	$=$	$-z_{0.99}$
$z_{0.025}$	$=$	1.96	$=$	$-z_{0.975}$
$z_{0.05}$	$=$	1.645	$=$	$-z_{0.95}$
$z_{0.10}$	$=$	1.28	$=$	$-z_{0.90}$
$z_{0.15}$	$=$	1.04	$=$	$-z_{0.85}$
$z_{0.20}$	$=$	0.84	$=$	$-z_{0.80}$

function (cdf) is denoted by $\Phi(z) = \Pr\{Z < z\}$. The upper $100 \times \alpha\%$ -tile of Φ is denoted by $z_\alpha = \Phi^{-1}(1 - \alpha) = -\Phi^{-1}(\alpha) = -z_{1-\alpha}$. Table 4.1 gives examples of z_α that are useful for common practice of statistics in clinical trials.

Under the alternative hypothesis, T is normally distributed with mean $\Delta\sqrt{\dfrac{n}{2\sigma^2}}$ and variance 1. The required sample size can be more conveniently derived by a one-sided test at the level of $\alpha/2$ as follows:

The type I error rate specification for the test is $\alpha/2 = \Pr(Z > c|H_0)$, which implies that the critical value $c = z_{\alpha/2} = -z_{1-\alpha/2}$. The desired power, by definition, is

$$1 - \beta = P(T > c|H_A) = P(T > z_{\alpha/2}|H_A)$$

$$= P\left(T - \Delta\sqrt{\frac{n}{2\sigma^2}} > z_{\alpha/2} - \Delta\sqrt{\frac{n}{2\sigma^2}} \,\middle|\, H_A \right)$$

$$= P\left(Z > z_{\alpha/2} - \Delta\sqrt{\frac{n}{2\sigma^2}} \right)$$

$$= 1 - \Phi\left(z_{\alpha/2} - \Delta\sqrt{\frac{n}{2\sigma^2}} \right)$$

This implies that

$$z_{\alpha/2} - \Delta\sqrt{\frac{n}{2\sigma^2}} = \Phi^{-1}(\beta) = -z_\beta \qquad (4.3)$$

Hence, we obtain

$$n = \frac{2\sigma^2\left(z_{\alpha/2} + z_\beta\right)^2}{\Delta^2} \qquad (4.4)$$

That is, we require a sample size of n in each treatment group to detect a mean difference of Δ with a power of $1-\beta$ by a one-sided test with type I error rate of $\alpha/2$. The same formula (Equation 4.4) applies to an evenly split α-level two-sided test $|T| > z_{\alpha/2}$ as well. This is because

$$P(|T| > z_{\alpha/2}) = P(T < -z_{\alpha/2}) + P(T > z_{\alpha/2}) \approx P(T > z_{\alpha/2})$$

where the first term is almost 0 under H_A. The form of Equation 4.4 will also be useful for other sample size calculations in the next few sections for different endpoints.

The power and alpha level are set more or less by convention (Table 4.1). The factors that are not preset and matter the most for estimating the required sample size are σ and Δ. The ratio of Δ/σ is the *standardized treatment difference*, which is also referred to as *(treatment) effect size*. Its reciprocal is the *coefficient of variation* σ/Δ. The power curve is a function of the sample size and the treatment effect size for a given trial. As shown in Equation 4.4, a smaller effect size Δ/σ (or, equivalently, a larger coefficient of variation) requires a larger sample size. A general idea for the magnitude of sample size is listed below for $\alpha/2 = 0.025$ and $1 - \beta = 0.80$:

$$\Delta/\sigma \approx 0.2 \text{ (small effect size) requires n} \approx 400$$
$$\approx 0.5 \text{ (medium effect size) requires n} \approx 70$$
$$\approx 0.8 \text{ (large effect size) requires n} \approx 25$$

In practice, one should review the literature or prior studies to obtain an idea of the control group's μ_2 and σ. If the control is a placebo, then the disease's natural history provides valuable background information. The project statistician should consult with the clinical investigator regarding a meaningful or expected treatment difference Δ. Note that clinical investigators often express expected treatment effect in terms of the relative change, $r = (\mu_1 - \mu_2)/\mu_2$ instead of the absolute change $\Delta = \mu_1 - \mu_2$. With the information on μ_2 and r, it is just a simple step to convert r to $\Delta = r\mu_2$.

Information regarding the within-group σ is more difficult to obtain. A homogeneous patient cohort will have a smaller σ, and from Equation 4.3 we can see that a smaller σ results in a smaller n (i.e., a more efficient design). However, a homogeneous cohort comes at the expense of limited generalizability to a wider, more heterogeneous population. A method to include a heterogeneous population while maintaining study efficiency is the stratified randomization design. With a stratified randomization, using a prognostic factor as a covariate in the analysis reduces the variance σ^2. (That is, it reduces the variance from marginal to conditional variance.) This fact also reminds us that, when using data from another study as a reference, we need to be sure to use the right *mean squared error* (MSE) from the ANOVA or ANCOVA (analysis of covariance) for an appropriate estimate of σ^2. Unfortunately, the medical literature usually publishes little information about variance. Sometimes we need to go several steps into a paper's summary table to find a useful estimate of the variance. For example, it sometimes is hidden in the confidence intervals. A recent medical paper by Puntoni et al. (2013) provides a good exercise (Homework 4.1).

Specifically, for a linear regression model (which includes ANOVA/ANCOVA) with several covariates expressed as

$$Y = \beta_0 + \beta_1 X_1 + \beta_2 X_2 + \dots + \beta_k X_K + e$$

the marginal variance of Y, $Var(Y) = \sigma_Y^2$ could be very large (this would induce a large, conservative sample size). The conditional variance (adjusted for covariates), $Var(Y|X) = Var(e) = \sigma_e^2$ might be more suitable for the sample size estimation formula (Equation 4.4), if the same covariates are used in the new trial as in the literature. Note that $\sigma_e^2 = (1 - R^2)\sigma_Y^2$, where R is the multiple correlation of the covariates with the outcome Y. The reduction of the variance depends on the prognostic importance of the covariates to the outcome Y. More discussion of ANCOVA is given in Chapter 5. Readers may want to review linear regression analysis (e.g., Weisberg 1985) as homework (Homework 4.2).

In practice, because investigators are often not certain about the effect size, it is useful to present a table or a power function graph for a range of sample sizes and possible effect sizes via Equation 4.5 when preparing a study proposal or trial protocol:

$$1 - \beta = \Phi\left(\sqrt{\frac{n}{2}} \frac{\Delta}{\sigma} - z_{\alpha/2} \right) \tag{4.5}$$

Example 4.1

A randomized trial was conducted to assess the effectiveness of Relenza, a new treatment for influenza, compared with placebo. The primary variable of interest was the number of days to alleviation of symptoms. A previous study suggested that a sensible value for σ was 2.75 days. The minimally clinically relevant difference, Δ, that the trial should have a good power to detect, was taken to be 1 day. The investigators used a significance level of $\alpha = 0.05$ (two-sided) and aimed for 90% power ($\beta = 0.1$). We calculate the sample size per group to meet these design parameters as follows:

$$n = \frac{2(z_{\alpha/2} + z_\beta)^2}{(\Delta/\sigma)^2} = \frac{2(1.96 + 1.28)^2}{(1/2.75)^2} = 158.8 \approx 160$$

Rounding the sample size up to a convenient integer is a common-sense practice for conservativeness. Sample size estimation is not exact mathematics because the design factors we assume (such as $\sigma = 2.75$) are approximations. Figure 4.1 presents a power curve for a range of alternative values $\Delta = \mu_1 - \mu_2$ for $n = 160$ per group. It is also informative to depict the power functions for different scenarios of sample size, as shown in Figure 4.2. When showing a power curve as a function of Δ, values of Δ are interpreted as detectable differences, for which the minimally clinically relevant difference is one of them with the targeted power.

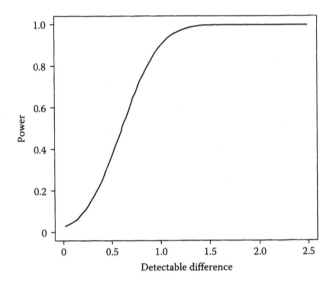

FIGURE 4.1
Power curve versus detectable $\Delta = \mu_1 - \mu_2$ for n = 160 per group.

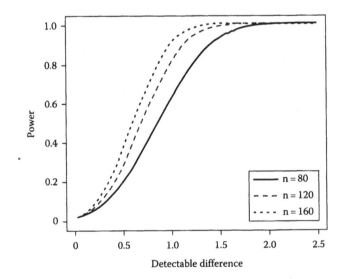

FIGURE 4.2
Power plot: Power versus detectable difference in means for different n.

4.3 Comparing Proportions for Binary Outcomes

For a randomized design with an equal allocation that compares two parallel treatment groups with a binary outcome, let $Y_i = 0$ or 1 ($= 1$ with probability π_i) for group $i = 1$ or 2. Without loss of generality, we let $Y = 1$ when observing an outcome event. The mean and variance parameters are

$$E(Y_i) = \pi_i$$

$$Var(Y_i) = \pi_i(1-\pi_i)$$

The treatment effect of interest may be the difference in the probability of an event in the two treatment groups: $\Delta = \pi_1 - \pi_2$. Other measures such as rate ratio π_1/π_2 or odds ratio $\pi_1(1 - \pi_2)/\pi_2(1 - \pi_1)$ are not considered in this section. The rate ratio can be transformed by taking the (natural) logarithm and the variance for the difference in the log scale can be found using the delta method. See Appendix 4.2 for the delta method. A method for odds ratio is included as a special case in Section 4.7. The null hypothesis of equal probability of the event occurring in both treatment groups is $H_0: \Delta = 0$ (Homework 4.3).

Sample estimates of the event probability π_1 and π_2 are proportions p_1 and p_2, respectively. Under H_0 ($\pi_1 = \pi_2$), the variance of $p_1 - p_2$ is

$$V_0 = \frac{2\bar{\pi}(1-\bar{\pi})}{n}$$

where $\bar{\pi} = (\pi_1 + \pi_2)/2$ is the average probability of event over the treatment groups.

Under H_A, the variance of $p_1 - p_2$ is

$$V_1 = \frac{\pi_1(1-\pi_1)+\pi_2(1-\pi_2)}{n}$$

There are two kinds of formulas given for tests of proportions in many introductory biostatistics books. One is

$$n = \frac{2\bar{\pi}(1-\bar{\pi})\left(z_{\alpha/2}+z_\beta\right)^2}{\Delta^2} \tag{4.6}$$

which is based on the *score test*. The derivation follows the same procedure as Equation 4.4 using the variance of $(p_1 - p_2)$ under H_0. (For the score test, the se in the denominator of Equation 4.2 is derived under the null hypothesis.)

The other formula is based on the *Wald test*, also derived from the same procedure as Equation 4.4 using the variance of $(p_1 - p_2)$ under H_0 and H_A:

$$n = \frac{\left(z_{\alpha/2}\sqrt{2\bar{\pi}(1-\bar{\pi})}+z_\beta\sqrt{\pi_1(1-\pi_1)+\pi_2(1-\pi_2)}\right)^2}{\Delta^2} \tag{4.7}$$

Again, n is the number of subjects required for each treatment group in order to detect a difference of at least Δ with power $(1-\beta) \times 100\%$ using a two-sided α level test. The Wald test and the score test are asymptotically equivalent, hence the n calculated from these two formulas should not be too different. The formula based on the score test is certainly simpler, thus it is also used in many other places, such as the group sequential design, as we see in Chapter 8.

4.4 Comparing Time-to-Event (Survival) Endpoints

4.4.1 Outcome Event

For a trial with time-to-event data, it is important to define the *outcome event*. Often the primary and the secondary endpoints refer to different sets of events. The event for the *overall survival* (OS) endpoint is death from any cause, that is, the event is all-cause mortality. For the endpoint of *progression-free survival* (PFS), both death and disease progression are counted as the outcome event, whichever occurs first. For the endpoint of *time to progression* (TTP), however, only disease progression is counted as the outcome event, whereas death prior to progression is considered a *censoring event*. TTP is used mostly in tumor recurrence studies. A good reference that discusses the merits of OS, PFS, and TTP in cancer trials is the FDA guidance document *Guidance for Industry: Clinical Trial Endpoints for the Approval of Cancer Drugs and Biologics* (CDER and CBER 2005). In cancer trials, determining disease progression in solid tumors involves measuring the tumor size physically or by radiologic images/scans and the radiologist's subjective assessment. How to standardize and maintain the quality of the progression assessment is an important issue of design and conduct for clinical trials with this type of data. Without ambiguity, we use the general term "survival" for all types of time-to-event variables in the following discussion.

4.4.2 Exponential Distribution Model with and without Censoring

Commonly used tests for comparing two time-to-event (survival) curves can be derived in several different ways: nonparametrically by combining a sequence of hypergeometric 2×2 tables, semiparametrically by using the partial likelihood function, or parametrically by assuming a distribution such as the exponential or the Weibull distribution model (see, e.g., Collett 1994). Some basic points of survival data analysis are given in Appendices 4.1–4.4 of this chapter. For a simple sample size calculation, the parametric approach is the easiest. In this section, we derive a formula for sample size under the exponential distribution without and with censoring.

Assume equal allocation of two treatment groups in a randomized trial. Let $y_{11}, \ldots, y_{1n}$ be the times to event in the test group; they are identically, independently distributed (iid) from the exponential distribution with the probability density function (pdf)

$$f_1(y) = \lambda_1 e^{\lambda_1 y}$$

and $y_{21}, \ldots, y_{2n}$ be the times to event in the control group; iid with pdf

$$f_2(y) = \lambda_2 e^{\lambda_2 y}$$

The parameter $\lambda > 0$ in the exponential model is called the *hazard rate*. With the exponential model, we explicitly assume that the hazard rate is a constant over time. First, let us assume no censoring, that is, everyone has an event, so that the event number d = n per treatment group, and the total event number is D = 2n = 2d. This is similar to assuming no missing data in the continuous or the binary case; actually, without censoring, this endpoint is also a continuous variable: time. The adjustment of randomly missing data in a continuous case or randomly censored data, in this case, is explained in Section 4.8.3.

We are interested in comparing the hazard rates between the two treatment groups. This is typically done by testing the log of the hazard ratios, log(HR). The null hypothesis of equal hazard rates is

$$H_0: \log(\lambda_1/\lambda_2) = 0$$

Let $\overline{Y}_1 = \sum_{1}^{n} y_{1i} / n$. The *maximum likelihood estimate* (MLE) of the hazard rate λ_1 and its asymptotic distribution is

$$\hat{\lambda}_1 = \frac{1}{\overline{Y}_1} \sim AN\left(\lambda_1, \frac{\lambda_1^2}{n}\right)$$

(See Appendix 4.2. The notation AN above stands for *asymptotic normal distribution*.) However, $\log(\hat{\lambda}_1)$ has a better approximation than $\hat{\lambda}_1$. Using the delta method, we can find the distribution of $\log(\hat{\lambda}_1)$:

$$\log(\hat{\lambda}_1) \sim N\left(\log\lambda_1, \frac{1}{n}\right) \tag{4.8}$$

The same is true for the hazard rate λ_2. (See Appendix 4.2 for the delta method.)

We then apply the same formula as in the continuous case (Equation 4.4), where Equation 4.8 corresponds to the form of $\overline{X} \sim N\left(\mu, \dfrac{\sigma^2}{n}\right)$. By switching parameters: $\Delta = \log(\lambda_1/\lambda_2)$ and $\sigma = 1$ (since $n = d$ without censoring), we have

$$d = \frac{2\left(Z_{\alpha/2} + Z_\beta\right)^2}{\Delta^2}$$

Or, as commonly used for a survival study, the total number of events:

$$D = \frac{4\left(Z_{\alpha/2} + Z_\beta\right)^2}{\Delta^2} \tag{4.9}$$

In Equation 4.9, we need to determine the value of $\Delta = \log(\lambda_1/\lambda_2)$. This is often accomplished by finding out the reference hazard rate, λ_2, from the literature and proposing a percent decrease for the test agent for λ_1. The medical literature often reports a landmark survival time (e.g., 5-year survival probability) or a median survival time (if reached). Because the cumulative survival function $S(y) = 1 - F(y)$, then for the exponential model,

$$S(y) = \exp(-\lambda y) \tag{4.10}$$

we can convert the landmark survival probability or the median survival time to the hazard rate (Homework 4.4). Table 4.2 lists survival summaries for three different exponential distribution models.

Equation 4.9 is simple in the sense that it unrealistically assumes no censoring and that all patients reach the endpoint (i.e., there is no definite study end time). Now, let us consider censoring in the following scenario:

Suppose that the random censoring time C (perhaps as a result of a competing risk such as adverse events in a time-to-pain-relief study or death in a TTP cancer study) is independent of the (outcome) event time

TABLE 4.2

Survival Summaries with Exponential Distribution Models

Hazard Rate (λ)	Mean Survival Time $(1/\lambda)$	Standard Deviation of Survival Time $(1/\lambda)$	Median Survival Time $((\log 2)/\lambda)$
1.5	0.67	0.67	0.46
1.0	1.00	1.00	0.69
0.5	2.00	2.00	1.39

and is also exponentially distributed with the same parameter η for both treatment groups. Then the probability of observing an outcome event in the test group during the study (of length L) is

$$P_1 = P(Y_1 < L, Y_1 < C) = \int_0^L \left[\int_u^\infty \eta e^{-\eta c} \, dc \right] \lambda_1 e^{-\lambda_1 u} \, du$$

$$= \frac{\lambda_1}{\lambda_1 + \eta} \left(1 - e^{-(\lambda_1 + \eta)L} \right) \tag{4.11}$$

Likewise,
$$P_2 = \frac{\lambda_2}{\lambda_2 + \eta} \left(1 - e^{-(\lambda_2 + \eta)L} \right)$$

With an equal allocation of patients, n, per group, the total expected number of events is

$$D = d_1 + d_2 = n(P_1 + P_2)$$

Hence, to adjust for censoring, we can first calculate D from Equation 4.9, and then the number of patients needed per group is

$$n = D/(P_1 + P_2) \tag{4.12}$$

The hazard rate of the censoring due to withdrawal, $\eta > 0$, has to be assumed as well for Equation 4.11. As for the hazard rate for the outcome event, one can assume a cumulative censoring rate and convert it to η. The case $\eta = 0$ reduces to the case where the censoring of outcome event is only due to the finite study end time L. That is, $P_i = P(Y_i < L) = 1 - e^{-\lambda_i L}$ for $i = 1, 2$ (Homework 4.5).

Alternatively, one can use the assumed cumulative censoring rate directly to make an adjustment. Section 4.8.1 uses this simple approach. Note that Equation 4.12 assumes that all patients are enrolled at time 0, which is not realistic in practice. However, the same formula applies to the more realistic case of random (right) censoring due to staggered entry of patients with the same study duration for each patient. When patients have different follow-up duration (e.g., early entries have longer follow-up than later entries for the same study end time), the entry pattern will determine the differential follow-up times, hence a more complicated formula involving entry distribution within recruitment time is needed. Further information about this topic is discussed in Chapter 9.

In addition, clinical trials with a time-to-event endpoint, especially when the event is fatal or life-threatening (myocardial infarction, stroke, cancer progression, etc.), usually involve group sequential designs with interim analyses. In Chapter 8, we cover the maximum sample size and expected sample size for group sequential trials. In Chapter 9, we discuss the monitoring of the maximum sample size.

4.4.3 Log-Rank Test under Weibull Distribution

The hazard rate under the exponential model is constant over time. Sometimes, the hazard rate may not be constant, but increasing or decreasing over time. In that case, it is a function of time, which can be denoted as h(t), and a Weibull distribution is a better choice of model. If a random variable $X \sim \exp(\lambda)$, then $Y = X^{1/k} \sim \text{Weibull}(\lambda, k)$. The parameter k (>0) controls how the hazard function h(t) varies with time (i.e., the shape of the hazard function). If $k > 1$, then the hazard is increasing with time; otherwise, if $0 < k < 1$, it is decreasing with time. For sample size calculation, one needs to first assume a value for this shape parameter (a common γ value for both treatment groups). To be specific, the hazard function of a Weibull(λ, k) is

$$h(t) = k\lambda^k t^{k-1} \tag{4.13}$$

and the survival distribution is

$$S(t) = e^{-(\lambda t)^k} \tag{4.14}$$

The null hypothesis can be expressed in terms of the median survival time:

$$m = [\log(2)]^{1/k}/\lambda \tag{4.15}$$

or, equivalently, in terms of transformed λ as

$$\theta = \lambda^k = \log(2)/m^k \tag{4.16}$$

That is, the null hypothesis is that the two treatment groups have equal median survival times or equal θ. Note that $Y^k = X$ is $\exp(\theta)$. Comparing Equation 4.14 to Equation 4.10, we find that for a specific k, if we regard $\theta = \lambda^k$ as the parameter of interest, with the transformed time t^k, then the model simplifies to the exponential model and we can utilize the result found there. From Equation 4.9, we obtain the needed total number of events:

$$D = \frac{4(Z_{\alpha/2} + Z_\beta)^2}{\Delta^2}$$

$$= \frac{4(Z_{\alpha/2} + Z_\beta)^2}{\left[\log\left(\dfrac{\theta_1}{\theta_2}\right)\right]^2} \tag{4.17}$$

where θ_1 and θ_2 are the median survival times m_1 and m_2, respectively, from Equation 4.16 for the two treatment groups under the alternative hypothesis.

4.4.4 Log-Rank Test under Proportional Hazards Model

The formulas in Equations 4.9 and 4.17 are based on parametric model assumptions. Semiparametrically, we can also work out a sample size formula for a general proportional hazards model as argued in the following, without going through mathematical details.

First, we note that whether the hazard rate is constant (as in the exponential model) or a function of time (as in the Weibull model), the null hypothesis uses the log of median survival times. The median survival time is a function of the parameter(s) that is (are) not a function of time. The proportional hazard model is a general setting, which says that the ratio of the hazards is a constant, although the hazards may change over time. Specifically, the general model is expressed as

$$h_1(t) = \varphi h_2(t) \qquad (4.18)$$

where $h_i(t)$ is the hazard function of the outcome event for the treatment group i, $i = 1, 2$. In terms of the survival function, it is

$$S_1(t) = [S_2(t)]^\varphi \qquad (4.19)$$

without specifying a parametric distribution.

The null hypothesis of interest is $\varphi = 1$, or $\log(\varphi) = 0$. The parameter φ is the *hazard ratio* (HR), where $\varphi = \lambda_1/\lambda_2$ for the exponential model, and $\varphi = \theta_1/\theta_2 = (\lambda_1/\lambda_2)^r$ for the Weibull model.

Using the large sample theory of the score statistic, one can derive the nonparametric version of the log-rank test. The general formula for the total number of events needed is the same as before:

$$D = \frac{4(Z_{\alpha/2} + Z_\beta)^2}{\Delta^2}$$

where Δ is the treatment effect expressed in the alternative hypothesis, which is the log of the hazard ratio, or $\log(HR) = \log(\varphi)$.

4.5 Clustered (or Correlated) Observations

In some clinical trials, *subunits* are clustered within the *main unit* (*cluster*). The treatment is randomized and administered to the main unit but measurements are taken on the subunit. Hence, the subunits nested within a main unit are correlated observations. Examples include the following:

- Dental studies, in which a tooth is the subunit, nested in a patient (main unit or cluster).
- A repeated measures design, where an observation at each time point is a subunit, nested in the subject.
- Community trials, such as trials on teaching methods, in which students are taught in classes. The class is the main unit and the students are the subunits nested in each class.

In a randomized trial that compares Group X versus Group Y with equal allocation, let the observations be denoted

$$Y_{ij}\, i = 1, \ldots , n \text{ (main unit)}; j = 1, \ldots , m_i \text{ (subunit)}$$

By design, we often set $m_i = m$ for all i so that all main units contain the same number of subunits. A random effect model is useful to induce the correlation among the subunits as follows: Let

$$Y_{ij} = \mu_i + e_{ij}; \mu_i \text{ and } e_{ij} \text{ are independent} \qquad (4.20)$$

with

$$E(\mu_i) = \mu_y, \operatorname{Var}(\mu_i) = \sigma_b^2 \text{ (between-cluster variability)}$$

$$E(e_{ij}) = 0, \operatorname{Var}(e_{ij}) = \sigma_w^2 \text{ (within-cluster, between-subunit variability)}$$

Therefore, the total variance of an observation Y_{ij} and the covariance between observations Y_{ij} and Y_{ik} within the ith cluster are

$$\operatorname{Var}(Y_{ij}) = \sigma^2 = \sigma_b^2 + \sigma_w^2$$

$$\operatorname{Cov}(Y_{ij}, Y_{ik}) = \operatorname{Var}(\mu_i) = \sigma_b^2$$

The correlation (corr) among subunits within a cluster equals

$$\rho = \frac{\sigma_b^2}{\sigma^2} \qquad (4.21)$$

This correlation is the same across all subunits and is called the *compound symmetry* model in the repeated measures context.

We model the data from group X the same way, except that $E(\mu_i) = \mu_x$ for clusters of X.

We now take advantage of the form of Equation 4.4 again. We first average over the subunits within each cluster i in the group Y and obtain $\overline{Y}_1$. Note that

$$E(\overline{Y}_{i\cdot}) = E(Y_{ij}) = \mu_Y$$

$$Var(\overline{Y}_{i\cdot}) = \frac{1}{m^2} Var\left(\sum_j Y_{ij}\right)$$

$$= \frac{1}{m^2}\left[Var(Y_{i1}) + ... + Var(Y_{im}) + Cov(Y_{i1}, Y_{i2}) + ... + Cov(Y_{i(m-1)}, Y_{im})\right]$$

$$= \frac{1}{m^2}\left[m\sigma^2 + m(m-1)\sigma_b^2\right] \tag{4.22}$$

$$= \frac{1}{m}\left[\sigma^2 + (m-1)\rho\sigma^2\right]$$

$$= \frac{1}{m}\left[1 + (m-1)\rho\right]\sigma^2$$

The same is true for group X.

We can see that in Equation 4.22 the mean of the cluster average remains an unbiased estimate of the population mean. However, the variance is modified by an extra multiplier, $1 + (m-1)\rho$, in comparison with the average of m independent samples. If $m > 1$ and $\rho > 0$, then there is an inflation of the variance due to the positive correlation among the subunits.

We next calculate the number of clusters needed per group (n) for testing $H_0\ \Delta = \mu_x - \mu_y = 0$, using the cluster averages as the observations. Plug the appropriate variance in Equation 4.22 into Equation 4.4 to obtain the following:

$$n = \frac{2\sigma^2\left[1 + (m-1)\rho\right](z_{\alpha/2} + z_\beta)^2}{m\Delta^2} \tag{4.23}$$

The total number of main units (clusters) equals $N = 2n$ and the total number of subunits (observations) equals $N \times m$.

If a pilot study is conducted to collect information for a future study with this kind of design, we would need to fit a *nested* ANOVA model (also called a *split-plot* model in the context of other *design of experiments*, or a simple random effect with compound symmetry model in a *repeated measures analysis*). Caution is required to identify the right MSE for the right variances for Equation 4.23. The following in-class exercise and homework assignment illustrate this point.

In-Class Exercise: Mental 2-Inch Experiment Students should first put away their rulers (note that rulers will be needed at a later point). Each student will be given a piece of paper and asked to draw a 2-inch segment on it without a ruler, write their initials on it, and hand in the piece of paper. After all papers have been collected, more blank sheets of paper will be distributed, and the students will be asked to again draw a 2-inch segment and mark their initials. All papers will again be collected, shuffled, and redistributed to the class, in such a way that no one receives their own papers or papers with the same initials. Students will then be asked to take out a ruler, measure the length of each segment, and record the length next to the segment. The length should be recorded in a standard fashion: (integer:a) + (integer:b)/16. Analyzing the collected data will be a homework assignment for the class (Homework 4.6).

This exercise has multiple purposes: (1) to illustrate the thought process of a statistical model to describe the data from an experiment; (2) to let readers practice some of the procedures in SAS for data analysis; (3) to find the variance estimates for sample size estimation for clustered (correlated) data; and (4) to construct a confidence interval to estimate the true mean, which is known (2 inches).

4.6 Sample Size for Testing a Noninferiority or Equivalence Hypothesis

The Helsinki Declaration (1976) published by the World Medical Association (WMA) has a mandate that all clinical research should avoid unnecessary suffering and injury and that, for a clinical trial, the investigator should make sure that there is no reasonable alternative to conducting the experiment. With the advancement of medicine in the last few decades, these ethical principles have now been updated by the WMA to include the consideration of avoiding the use of placebo as the control in a clinical trial whenever there is a standard medical practice available to treat the disease with an approved active medicine. Many clinical trials use an add-on design that includes having the placebo and the test drug added to the standard care. There are also trials that compare the test compound head-to-head with an active control that has been approved and used in practice. In the latter scenario, the hypothesis of superiority may require an unaffordable sample size to detect a miniscule improvement. In this case, a common approach is to test the null hypothesis of inferiority and the alternative hypothesis of noninferiority within a designated margin of acceptance for the test compound compared to the active control. In the meantime, the trial also has the purpose of showing that the new compound has other advantages such as lower cost, more convenient administration, better safety profile, etc.

For a noninferiority trial, the first step is to establish a margin, $\delta > 0$, to define the boundary between inferiority and noninferiority. For the case of continuous endpoints where a greater value implies a better outcome and the mean difference is $\Delta = \mu_x - \mu_y$, the set up of hypotheses is

H_0: $\Delta < -\delta$ (implying X is inferior to Y by more than $-\delta$ from the mean)

H_A: $\Delta \geq -\delta$ (implying X is NOT inferior to Y by more than $-\delta$ from the mean)

This is a one-sided test. It is convenient to carry out an α-level test by constructing a one-sided $(1-\alpha) \times 100\%$ confidence interval (CI) for $\Delta = \mu_x - \mu_y$. We reject H_0 when the lower bound of the $(1-\alpha) \times 100\%$ CI is greater than $-\delta$, as shown in Figure 4.3:

The power of this test is equal to

$$P\left(\hat{\Delta} - z_\alpha se\left(\hat{\Delta}\right) \geq -\delta \mid -\delta \leq \Delta\right) = 1 - \beta \qquad (4.24)$$

Usually we pick a specific value for Δ in the H_A space, say $\Delta = \Delta^* > -\delta$, to achieve a desired power. Then

$$\hat{\Delta} - \Delta^* = \overline{X} - \overline{Y} - \Delta^* \sim N\left(0, \frac{2\sigma^2}{n}\right)$$

and

$$\left(\hat{\Delta} - \Delta^*\right) - z_\alpha se\left(\hat{\Delta}\right) \geq -\delta - \Delta^* \text{ if and only if } \frac{\left(\overline{X} - \overline{Y}\right) - \Delta^*}{\sqrt{\frac{2\sigma^2}{n}}} \geq z_\alpha - \frac{\left(\delta + \Delta^*\right)}{\sqrt{\frac{2\sigma^2}{n}}}$$

FIGURE 4.3
Graphical representation of a noninferiority test.

From Equation 4.24 and the assumption of $\Delta = \Delta^*$, we have

$$-z_\beta = z_\alpha - \frac{(\delta + \Delta^*)}{\sqrt{\dfrac{2\sigma^2}{n}}}$$

which leads to

$$n = \frac{2\sigma^2 (z_\alpha + z_\beta)^2}{(\delta + \Delta^*)^2} \tag{4.25}$$

for all $\Delta^* > -\delta$.

For testing the equivalence hypotheses, H_0: $|\Delta| \geq \delta$ (nonequivalence) versus H_A: $|\Delta| < \delta$ (equivalence), we would construct a two-sided $(1 - 2\alpha) \times 100\%$ confidence interval for Δ to see if the CI falls entirely within $(-\delta, \delta)$. For the sample size and power calculation, we may set $\Delta = \Delta^* = 0$ for the alternative hypothesis (as being "truly" equivalent). Comparing this hypothesis to the two-sided hypothesis situation in Section 4.2, the only difference is that the null and the alternative hypotheses are switched. Therefore, we only need to switch the type I and type II errors in Equation 4.4 to obtain the sample size per group for a power of $1 - \beta$ in this situation:

$$n = \frac{2\sigma^2 (z_{\beta/2} + z_\alpha)^2}{\delta^2} \tag{4.26}$$

The above heuristic argument can be formally derived as shown in the following text. The resemblance of Equations 4.25 and 4.26 to Equation 4.4 highlights the role of the (non-) inferiority margin δ.

$$\alpha = P(\text{Reject } |\Delta| \geq \delta \mid |\Delta| \geq \delta)$$

$$= P(|T| < c \mid |\Delta| \geq \delta) \text{ where } T \sim N\left(\Delta\sqrt{\frac{n}{2\sigma^2}},\ 1\right)$$

$$\leq P(|T| < c \mid |\Delta| = \delta)$$

If $\Delta = \delta$ $\quad \alpha \leq P(T < c \mid \Delta = \delta) - P(T < -c \mid \Delta = \delta)$

$$= P\left(T - \delta\sqrt{\frac{n}{2\sigma^2}} < c - \delta\sqrt{\frac{n}{2\sigma^2}} \,\middle|\, \Delta = \delta\right) - P\left(T - \delta\sqrt{\frac{n}{2\sigma^2}} < -c - \delta\sqrt{\frac{n}{2\sigma^2}} \,\middle|\, \Delta = \delta\right)$$

$$\leq P\left(T - \delta\sqrt{\frac{n}{2\sigma^2}} < c - \delta\sqrt{\frac{n}{2\sigma^2}} \,\middle|\, \Delta = \delta\right) \quad \text{(the second positive term} \approx 0)$$

$$= P\left(Z < c - \delta\sqrt{\frac{n}{2\sigma^2}}\right)$$

Hence, $z_{1-\alpha} = c - \delta\sqrt{\dfrac{n}{2\sigma^2}}$, $c = -z_\alpha + \delta\sqrt{\dfrac{n}{2\sigma^2}}$.

That is, we reject H_0 when $T < -z_\alpha + \delta\sqrt{\dfrac{n}{2\sigma^2}}$.

If $\Delta = -\delta$ $\quad \alpha \le P(T < c \mid \Delta = -\delta) - P(T < -c \mid \Delta = -\delta)$

$$= P\left(T + \delta\sqrt{\frac{n}{2\sigma^2}} < c + \delta\sqrt{\frac{n}{2\sigma^2}} \mid \Delta = -\delta\right) - P\left(T + \delta\sqrt{\frac{n}{2\sigma^2}} < -c + \delta\sqrt{\frac{n}{2\sigma^2}} \mid \Delta = -\delta\right)$$

$$= P\left(Z < c + \delta\sqrt{\frac{n}{2\sigma^2}}\right) - P\left(Z < -c + \delta\sqrt{\frac{n}{2\sigma^2}}\right) \le 1 - P\left(Z < -c + \delta\sqrt{\frac{n}{2\sigma^2}}\right)$$

(the first term is ≈ 1)

$$= P\left(Z \ge -c + \delta\sqrt{\frac{n}{2\sigma^2}} \mid \Delta = -\delta\right)$$

Hence, $z_\alpha = -c + \delta\sqrt{\dfrac{n}{2\sigma^2}}$, $c = -z_\alpha + \delta\sqrt{\dfrac{n}{2\sigma^2}}$.

That is, we reject H_0 when $T \ge -z_\alpha + \delta\sqrt{\dfrac{n}{2\sigma^2}}$.

Note that the above shows that the two-sided $(1 - 2\alpha) \times 100\%$ CI approach is equivalent to rejecting H_0 (nonequivalence) when $|T| > -z_\alpha + \delta\sqrt{\dfrac{n}{2\sigma^2}}$. (Note that when n is large enough, $-z_\alpha + \delta\sqrt{\dfrac{n}{2\sigma^2}}$ is always positive.)

The power function is

$$g(\Delta) = P\left(T < -z_\alpha + \delta\sqrt{\frac{n}{2\sigma^2}} \text{ or } T \ge -z_\alpha + \delta\sqrt{\frac{n}{2\sigma^2}} \mid |\Delta| < \delta\right).$$

Set power $= 1 - \beta$ at $\Delta = 0$,

$$1 - \beta = P\left(T < -z_\alpha + \delta\sqrt{\frac{n}{2\sigma^2}} \text{ or } T \ge -z_\alpha + \delta\sqrt{\frac{n}{2\sigma^2}} \mid \Delta = 0\right) \text{ implies}$$

$$P\left(T \ge -z_\alpha + \delta\sqrt{\frac{n}{2\sigma^2}}\right) = \beta/2$$

Hence, $-z_\alpha + \delta\sqrt{\dfrac{n}{2\sigma^2}} = z_{\beta/2}$. This leads to Equation 4.26.

Example 4.2[*]

Two inhalers, A and B, used for the relief of asthma attacks, are to be assessed for equivalence. They will be considered equivalent if the two-sided 90% CI for the treatment difference measured by the morning peak expiratory flow rate (liter/min) falls entirely within the range of +/– 15 liter/min. That is, $\delta = 15$. From a previous trial the prior estimate of σ^2, the between-subject variance, is 1600 (liter/min)^2. We would like to claim equivalence, if they in fact are identical, with 80% power. From Table 4.1, we use $z_\alpha = z_{0.05} = 1.645$, $z_{\beta/2} = z_{0.10} = 1.28$ in Equation 4.26 to obtain:

$$n = \frac{2 \times 1600 \times (1.645 + 1.28)^2}{15^2} \approx 122$$

Each group should include 122 patients. If we construct a 95% CI for the equivalence test, then $z_\alpha = z_{0.025} = 1.96$, and $n \approx 150$.

4.7 Comparing Ordinal Endpoints by Wilcoxon–Mann–Whitney Test

Ordinal endpoints in clinical trials are usually used for quality of life questionnaires such as the short form SF-36 (Fayers and Machin 2000). When there are many (say, five or more) categories, one can assign a score to each category and treat the change from the baseline of the score as a continuous variable, then apply Equation 4.4 for the sample size calculation. Otherwise, using methods for ordered categorical data would be more appropriate. The Wilcoxon–Mann–Whitney (WMW) test, also known as the two-sample Wilcoxon rank-sum test (Wilcoxon 1945; Mann and Whitney 1947) is a popular method to compare two distributions $F(x)$ and $G(y)$ for two independent treatment groups. Because there is no specification of the shape and form of these distributions, it is a nonparametric test. The general null hypothesis is that the two distributions are the same. In the case of a continuous endpoint, any difference between distributions implies that $P(X < Y)$ no longer equals 1/2. Therefore, the WMW test is often also used to test the null hypothesis of $P(X < Y) = 1/2$. When ties exist (which is the case for ordinal data), $P(X = Y) \neq 0$, so we split the ties between $P(X < Y)$ and $P(X > Y)$. The null hypothesis would then be

$$P(X < Y) + 0.5P(X = Y) = 1/2$$

If one wants to test a specific aspect of the distributions such as $E(X) = E(Y)$, which is true if $F(x) = G(y)$, against $E(X) \neq E(Y)$, assuming

---

[*] From Jones, B., et al., *British Medical Journal*, 313, 36–39, 1996.

means exist, then we need to add the following assumption: If there is a difference between the two distributions, then it is in the location shift. That is, $F(x) = G(y + c)$, where c is some nonzero constant. However, when the outcome is bounded, as in the case of ordinal data presented in a contingency table, this shift hypothesis is not applicable. McCullagh (1980) suggested using the odds ratio (OR) as the effect size with the assumption of a proportional odds model. (In Section 4.4.4, we discussed the use of the semiparametric log-rank test under the proportional hazard model for comparing two survival distributions.) With fewer ordered categories (typically, no more than five), the proportional odds assumption is more likely to hold.

Specifically, suppose the outcome measure of interest has J ordered categories, $j = 1, \ldots, J$. Let π_{jX} be the probability of being in category j for a subject in treatment group X and $\Pi_{jX} = \sum_{i=1}^{j} \pi_{iX}$ be the (cumulative) probability of being in category j or less in group X. (Note that $\Pi_{JX} = 1$.) Likewise, assume π_{jY} and Π_{jY} for the control group Y. π_{j+} is the marginal probability of category j. The proportional odds assumption states that

$$OR_j = \frac{\Pi_{jX}(1 - \Pi_{jY})}{\Pi_{jY}(1 - \Pi_{jX})} \text{ is the same } (OR_j = OR) \quad \text{for all } j = 1, \ldots, J-1$$

The null hypothesis in terms of OR is

$$H_0: OR = 1 \text{ or } \log(OR) = 0$$

By specifying a particular OR value for the alternative hypothesis and assuming values for $\pi_{jX}\ j = 1, \ldots, J$ (if X is the control group), we have

$$\Pi_{jY} = \frac{\Pi_{jX}}{OR(1 - \Pi_{jX}) + \Pi_{jX}}, \quad j = 1, \ldots, J-1$$

Then, π_{jY} for each category $j = 1, \ldots, J$ can be calculated. Finally, the marginal probability π_{j+} of category j is obtained for each $j = 1$ to J. Whitehead (1993) provided a formula of sample size per group:

$$n = \frac{6(Z_{\alpha/2} + Z_\beta)^2}{OR^2\left(1 - \sum_{j=1}^{J} \pi_{j+}^3\right)} \tag{4.27}$$

Equation 4.27 is given here without derivation. There is a homework assignment to compare Equation 4.27 with the result based on simulation of the WMW test (Homework 4.7).

4.8 Sample Size Adjustments

4.8.1 Adjustment for Loss to Follow-Up

In almost all clinical trials some subjects are *lost to follow-up*, that is, they fail to complete the study and cannot be traced for their outcomes. The data lost will affect the study power. A possible problem that is more serious is that the missing data will also bias the result. We discuss this possibility in more detail in Chapter 10. Here we make an important assumption that the missing data from loss to follow-up are *missing at random* (MAR). MAR will be precisely defined in Chapter 10, but this essentially assumes that the missing data only affects the power and does not result in bias for the result.

Suppose r is the *projected* proportion of subjects that are lost to follow-up in the trial, and N is the total number of subjects necessary to recruit, taking into account loss to follow-up. With loss to follow-up, N^* is the number of patients available for analysis at the completion of the trial, based upon which we would like to detect a significant treatment effect with a desirable power.

We first use the formulas in the above sections to obtain the appropriate unadjusted sample size N^*. Then the sample size adjusted for the possible loss to follow-up is simply

$$N = N^*/(1 - r) \qquad (4.28)$$

The same applies to random right-censoring for the survival time case.

4.8.2 Adjustment for Nonadherence/Noncompliance

In almost all clinical trials, subjects sometimes fail to adhere to their assigned treatment regimen. This is also called a noncompliance issue. For example, in an open label active control study, because the active control agent is already approved and available in the market, it is possible for a patient to stop the experimental treatment and take the active control treatment if the patient feels the test treatment is not working well for him or her. Another possible scenario is that in a placebo-controlled trial, patients receiving the test treatment may discontinue the assigned treatment and leave untreated because of some intolerable side effect. Although medical principles mandate that subjects in a clinical trial may withdraw from the study treatment at will at any time and the investigator has the obligation to withdraw the subject for any foreseeable risk, the study protocol should be designed in such a way that the these patients' condition can still be followed up on, so that their outcome and other useful data can still be collected. The *intention-to-treat* (ITT) principle states that patients' data should be analyzed according to the original treatment group to which they were randomized and that all patients should be accounted for in an ITT analysis.

To understand the impact of noncompliance, we use the continuous outcome in a randomized trial of two treatment groups for illustration. This method is similar to other types of outcomes. Assume the true treatment means are μ_1 and μ_2. Let p be the proportion of subjects who are assigned to treatment group A but take Treatment B, and let q be the proportion of subjects who are assigned to treatment group B but take Treatment A. Under nonadherence, the resulting treatment means become

$$\mu_1^* = (1 - p)\mu_1 + p\mu_2$$

$$\mu_2^* = q\mu_1 + (1 - q)\mu_2$$

$$\text{Then, } \mu_1^* - \mu_2^* = (1 - p - q)(\mu_1 - \mu_2) \tag{4.29}$$

This treatment difference in Equation 4.29 should be used as the detectable treatment effect in the sample size calculation. We can see that $\mu_1^* - \mu_2^* \leq \mu_1 - \mu_2$. Hence, the required sample size will need to be larger to take into account the possible noncompliance.

4.8.3 Adjustment for Loss to Follow-Up and Nonadherence/Noncompliance

The combined impact of loss to follow-up and noncompliance on the required sample size can be calculated for a range of possible loss-to-follow-up proportion r and noncompliance proportions p and q. This impact is calculated by first making the adjustment described in Section 4.8.2, followed by the adjustment described in Section 4.8.1 (Equation 4.28).

4.8.4 Adjustment for Multiple Testing

The issue of multiple hypothesis testing can have different appearances, such as multiple endpoints or objectives, multiple treatment groups, multiple time points, and multiple (interim) analyses. For a clinical trial, especially a Phase III confirmatory trial, the FDA, EMA (European Medicines Agency), and health authorities in other regions require that the overall (family-wise) type I error rate be maintained, at most, at the 5% level for a two-sided test. Although there are more efficient ways to deal with the issue in the data analysis, for sample size calculation, the *Bonferroni correction* is considered the simplest and most conservative method to control the family-wise error rate. That is, we simply replace the type I error rate α in the above formulas with α/k, where k is the number of statistical tests that contribute to the claims on the label of the medication. This correction will dramatically increase the sample size if k is large. Therefore, it is advisable for a Phase III trial to have a limited number of objectives, endpoints, and treatment group comparisons.

4.9 Sample Size by Simulation and Bootstrap

In some situations when it is not straightforward to derive a sample size or power function formula by conventional methods, we can use computer simulations to estimate the sample size or plot the power function. An illustration is given in Homework 4.7 with the Wilcoxon rank-sum test, which is the most popular nonparametric test when the outcome is ordinal with a limited number of categories. This test is also popular in cases where the outcome is continuous with a very skewed distribution, while data transformation is undesirable for interpretation and the trial size is not large enough for applying the central limit theorem to the mean. In a simulation study for sample size and power estimation, data are generated and test statistics are calculated from the given models under the null as well the alternative hypotheses. If a reliable pilot data set is available, one can try anticipating the outcome of the trial by bootstrapping (repeated sampling with replacement) based on the available pilot data. Simulation and bootstrapping are very useful tools for design, development of methods, and analyses in clinical trials. See Tsodikove, Hasenclever, and Loeffler (1998) for an example in a chronic myelogenous leukemia trial, and Walters and Campbell (2005) for trials with health-related quality of life outcomes.

Appendix 4.1: Fundamentals of Survival Data Analysis

Survival distribution is the probability that an individual is event-free, "survives," to a certain time, t:

$$S(t) = Pr(T > t) = 1 - Prob(T \le t) = 1 - F(t)$$

If the time-to-event random variable T has an exponential distribution with the parameter $\lambda > 0$, then (Figure 4.4)

$$S(t) = \int_{T=t}^{\infty} f(T)dT = \int_{t}^{\infty} \lambda e^{-\lambda T} dT = e^{-\lambda t}$$

Hazard function is the instantaneous event rate that the given individual has survived to that point in time:

$$\lambda(t) = \lim_{\delta \to 0} \frac{Pr(t < T < t + \delta \mid T > t)}{\delta} = \frac{f(t)}{S(t)}$$

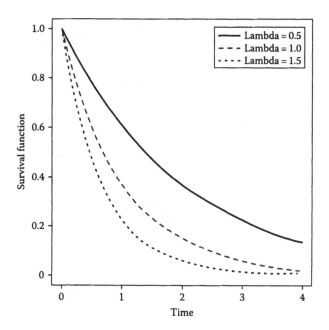

FIGURE 4.4
Survival function with exponential distribution models.

For exponential T, $\lambda(t) = \lambda$, and the expected failure time for an individual is

$$E(T) = \int_{t=0}^{\infty} tf(t)dt = \int_{0}^{\infty} t\lambda e^{-\lambda t} dt = \frac{1}{\lambda}$$

Appendix 4.2: Exponential Distribution Model

In the following, we continue to use the simple exponential distribution $\exp(\lambda)$ for summaries of basic concepts.

Likelihood:

$$L(\lambda; t_1, \ldots t_n) = \prod_{i=1}^{n} f(t_i) = \prod_{i=1}^{n} \lambda e^{-\lambda t_i} = \lambda^n \prod_{i=1}^{n} e^{-\lambda t_i}$$

Log-likelihood:

$$l(\lambda) = n \log \lambda - \lambda \sum_{i=1}^{n} t_i$$

MLE maximizes the (log-) likelihood. It is derived by taking the derivative of the log-likelihood with respect to λ, setting the resulting score function equal to 0 and solving for λ.

The derivative of the log-likelihood is called *score*: $\dfrac{n}{\lambda} - \displaystyle\sum_{i=1}^{n} t_i$

MLE: The solution of the score function is MLE, $\hat{\lambda} = \dfrac{n}{\displaystyle\sum_{i=1}^{n} t_i} = \dfrac{1}{t}$

The variance of the MLE is estimated as the inverse of the *Fisher information*:

$$I(\lambda) = -E_\lambda \left[\frac{\partial^2}{\partial \lambda^2} l(\lambda) \right]$$

Fisher information:

$$I(\lambda) = -E_\lambda \left[\frac{\partial^2}{\partial \lambda^2} l(\lambda) \right] = E_\lambda \left[\frac{n}{\lambda^2} \right] = \frac{n}{\lambda^2}$$

Therefore, $\quad \text{Var}\left[\hat{\lambda} \right] = \dfrac{\lambda^2}{n}$

Statistical theory shows that for all practical purposes, with a suitably large sample size, the MLE is normally distributed and unbiased. Thus,

$$\hat{\lambda} = \frac{1}{t} \sim \text{AN}\left(\lambda, \frac{\lambda^2}{n} \right)$$

The notation AN stands for *asymptotic normal distribution*.

Example 4.3

Suppose that in a study of chemoradiotherapy for patients with pancreatic cancer, the average survival time among 20 patients was found to be 15.1 months. We can calculate the 95% CI for the hazard around the point estimate of 1/15.1 (=0.066) deaths per month.

$$\left(\hat{\lambda} - z_{1-\alpha/2} \times \frac{\hat{\lambda}}{\sqrt{n}}, \ \hat{\lambda} + z_{1-\alpha/2} \times \frac{\hat{\lambda}}{\sqrt{n}} \right)$$

$$= \left(\frac{1}{15.1} - 1.96 \times \frac{1}{15.1\sqrt{20}}, \ \frac{1}{15.1} + 1.96 \times \frac{1}{15.1\sqrt{20}} \right)$$

$$= (0.037,\ 0.095)$$

Delta method: If $X \sim \text{AN}(\mu, V(X))$, then $g(X) \sim \text{AN}(g(\mu), g'(\mu)^2\, V(X))$ for continuous and differentiable function g.

$$\text{For } \hat{\lambda} \sim \text{AN}\left(\lambda, \frac{\lambda^2}{n}\right), \text{ then } \frac{1}{n}\sum_{i=1}^{n} t_i = \frac{1}{\hat{\lambda}} \sim \text{AN}\left(\frac{1}{\lambda}, (-\lambda^{-2})^2 \frac{\lambda^2}{n}\right) = \text{AN}\left(\frac{1}{\lambda}, \frac{1}{n\lambda^2}\right)$$

$$\text{and } \log(\hat{\lambda}) \sim \text{AN}\left(\log(\lambda), \left(\frac{1}{\lambda}\right)^2 \frac{\lambda^2}{n}\right) = \text{AN}\left(\log(\lambda), \frac{1}{n}\right).$$

Appendix 4.3: Survival with Independent Censoring

A censoring event should be distinguished from an outcome event. The outcome event is the primary interest. The censoring event might be some competing risk, which truncates the time to the outcome event when occurring before the outcome event. Without a competing risk, the fixed finite study duration could also censor the outcome event. Because the time scale starts at the origin (time zero) and extends to the right, this censoring due to a fixed study end time is usually called "right censoring."

Right censoring may happen in two possible ways: (1) All patients enter the study simultaneously and complete the study at the same calendar time; or more likely (2) patients enter and end the study at different calendar times but are followed up with the same duration of time. The study ends completely after the last patient completes the study. If an event has not occurred for a subject by his/her study end time, all we can say is that his/her time to event is greater than the observed follow-up time.

Notation

Y_i = time of event for subject i

C_i = time of censoring for subject i

$T_i = \min(Y_i, C_i)$

$\delta_i = 1$ if event was observed (i.e., $C_i > Y_i$)

$\quad = 0$ if censored at time C_i before event was observed (i.e., if $C_i < Y_i$)

The observed data: T_i and δ_i

Appendix 4.4: MLE with Censoring under the Exponential Model

Likelihood:

$$L(\lambda; t_1, \ldots t_n) = \prod_{i: \delta_i = 1} f(t_i) \prod_{i: \delta_i = 0} S(t_i)$$

$$= \prod_{i=1}^{n} \left[\lambda e^{-\lambda t_i} \right]^{\delta_i} \left[e^{-\lambda t_i} \right]^{1-\delta_i}$$

$$= \prod_{i=1}^{n} \lambda^{\delta_i} e^{-\lambda t_i}$$

Log-likelihood:

$$l(\lambda) = \left(\sum_{i=1}^{n} \delta_i \right) \log \lambda - \lambda \sum_{i=1}^{n} t_i = D \log \lambda - \lambda \sum_{i=1}^{n} t_i$$

Score equation:

$$\frac{D}{\lambda} - \sum_{i=1}^{n} t_i = 0$$

where D is total outcome events and $\sum_{i=1}^{n} t_i$ is the total follow-up time.

MLE: $\hat{\lambda} = \dfrac{D}{\sum\limits_{i=1}^{n} t_i}$

Fisher information:

$$I(\lambda) = -E\left[\frac{\partial^2}{\partial \lambda^2} l(\lambda) \right] = E\left[\frac{D}{\lambda^2} \right] = \frac{n\left(1 - e^{-\lambda C}\right)}{\lambda^2}$$

since $E(D) = nP(\delta_i = 1) = nP(Y_i < C_i) = n(1 - e^{-\lambda C})$ when all $C_i = C$ (i.e., all patients are subject to the same study duration C).

Therefore,

$$Var(\hat{\lambda}) = \frac{\lambda^2}{n\left(1 - e^{-\lambda C}\right)} = \frac{\lambda^2}{E(D)}$$

Homework 4.1

Study the paper "A Randomized, Placebo-Controlled, Preoperative Trial of Allopurinol in Subjects with Colorectal Adenoma" (Puntoni, M., et al., *Cancer Prevention Research*, 2013, 6: 74–81) and do the following:

1. Find the primary endpoint. Comment on Table 1 in light of our discussion in Chapter 2.

2. Do your own sample size calculation for this study: Set up the null and alternative hypotheses; define your notation, alpha, and power; and list all the necessary parameters, just as if you were the statistician of that project and were writing the study design in the protocol. The paper might not have all the necessary information explicitly written. You should derive information as needed. Compare your results with their calculation. (Hint: You may need to convert the relative change to absolute change and also find information regarding σ from the 95% CIs in their Table 2.)

3. Assume that the loss-to-follow-up rate is 15% and the nonadherence rate is 5% for one group and 3% for the other group. How many total patients do you then need to recruit for the study?

4. Write a SAS or R program for the above sample size calculation, make a "power curve plot" (i.e., power versus detectable delta/treatment effect) for three different sample sizes of your own choice to show the sensitivity of power versus n, just like Figure 4.2.

5. Note that the above exercise is like "playing detective" to guess "what happened when that study was planned" from the manuscript. Also note that this study was not a positive study. Suppose that later, researchers want to conduct another study of this kind, and ask you to use the results in this study as a reference to plan a new study. What would you recommend for the (revised) sample size for this new study?

Homework 4.2

Review the multiple linear regression formula $\sigma_e^2 = \left(1 - R^2\right)\sigma_Y^2$ from a linear regression textbook. Interpret the R^2.

Homework 4.3

The relative treatment effect for a binary outcome may also be measured by the ratio of event probabilities in the two treatment groups: $\Delta = \pi_1 / \pi_2$. Form the hypothesis test and obtain the sample size per group using the log transformation and delta method.

Homework 4.4

With an exponential model, $S(t) = \exp(-\lambda t)$. Show that the median survival time $m = \log(2)/\lambda$. With a Weibull(λ, γ) model, show that the median survival time is $m = [\log(2)]^{1/\gamma}/\lambda$.

Homework 4.5

A randomized clinical trial was planned to examine whether the glucocorticoid prednisone could prolong life relative to an inactive placebo treatment for patients with histologically verified liver cirrhosis. Historical data suggests that, when untreated, 50% of patients with liver cirrhosis die within 4.2 years. Estimate how many patients are needed to attain 90% power to test the null hypothesis of no effect of hormone at the 0.05 significance level when the treatment can increase median survival time by 0.5 years, 1 year, 1.5 years, 2 years, or 2.5 years (five scenarios).

1. Assume the exponential model with no censoring in the problem above and use the $\log(HR)$ as the effect size of interest. Organize all of the results in a single table of required sample sizes and comment on these results.

2. Consider terminating the observation of each individual after they have been followed up for 4, 6, 10 years (three different scenarios). Use the $\log(HR)$ as the effect size/estimate of interest. Organize all of these results as well as the results under no censoring in a single table of required sample sizes and provide an interpretation of and comment on these results. How much will the sample sizes be inflated to account for this censoring?

Homework 4.6

Referring to the "Mental 2-Inch Mini Experiment" (Section 4.5) conducted in class:

1. Discuss briefly how the data of the experiment can be modeled by Equation 4.20. What are the model parameters and what process when generating the data ensures the assumptions?

2. Input the data collected from n = 15 students into SAS; obtain estimates of the within-subject variance, the between-subject variance, and the population true value we are trying to estimate (here, we know the true value = 2 inches); and calculate the correlation between the first and second within-subject repeated measures.

Data

Student	Sequence	Measurement (inch)	Student	Sequence	Measurement (inch)
1	1	1.375	9	1	2.125
	2	1.375		2	2.0625
2	1	1.5625	10	1	1.625
	2	1.5		2	1.25
3	1	1.1875	11	1	2.28125
	2	1.175		2	2.4375
4	1	1.375	12	1	2
	2	1.25		2	2.375
5	1	2.46875	13	1	1.875
	2	2.34375		2	1.875
6	1	2.46875	14	1	1.5625
	2	2.3125		2	1.625
7	1	1.625	15	1	1.8125
	2	1.625		2	1.8125
8	1	2.0625			
	2	1.9375			

3. Verify that the within-class correlation obtained from Equation 4.21 matches the *Pearson correlation* from PROC CORR in SAS for paired data. Prove the theoretical equivalence of these two representations of correlation.

4. Part (b) may be performed in the following different ways available in SAS:

    a. Use a variance component model in PROC VARCOMP
    b. Use a model in PROC ANOVA
    c. Use a model in PROC GLM
    d. Use a random effect model in PROC MIXED

Treating this experiment as a pilot study for obtaining information of a control group to be used for a main study, use each of these above procedures in SAS to find the right estimate for the variances needed for a sample size calculation for the main trial with the same clustered/correlated measures.

Homework 4.7

Carry out simulations to calculate power and sample size for the WMW test for testing the general null hypothesis of identical distributions and compare the result with that from Equation 4.27 with the proportional odds alternative hypothesis.

Data: Let x_i ($i = 1, \ldots , n$) be random samples from population $F(x)$ and y_j ($j = 1, \ldots , m$) be random samples from population $G(y)$. Assign the ranks 1 to $N = n + m$ to them together. Let $R(x_i)$ denote the rank assigned to x_i and $R(y_j)$ be the rank assigned to y_j.

The WMW test statistic and critical value: If there are no ties, or just a few ties, the sum of the ranks assigned to treatment group X can be used as a test statistic:

$$T = \sum_i^n R(x_i)$$

For n or m greater than 20, the pth quantile w_p of T is approximated by

$$w_p = n(N+1)/2 + z_p\sqrt{nm(N+1)/12}$$

Thus, we reject the null hypothesis of identical distributions at alpha level, α, if $T > w_{1-\alpha}$. If there are many ties, then we use:

$$T_1 = \frac{\sum_i^n R(x_i) - n(N+1)/2}{\sqrt{\dfrac{nm}{N(N-1)}\sum_i^N R_i^2 - \dfrac{nm(N+1)^2}{4(N-1)}}}$$

where $\sum_{i=1}^N R_i^2$ refers to the sum of the squares of all N of the ranks or average ranks actually used in both samples. T_1 is approximately $N(0,1)$ under the null hypothesis of identical distributions for n or m greater than 20.

Simulate the power for the WMW test as follows:

1. We should first verify the test gives the correct type I error level. Generate $n = m = 50$ observations from two identical ordinal distributions (with four categories c1, c2, c4, and c6):

   $P(X = c1) = P(Y = c1) = 0.05$, $P(X = c2) = P(Y = c2) = 0.30$, $P(X = c4) = P(Y = c4) = 0.25$, and $P(X = c6) = P(Y = c6) = 0.40$

Calculate the test T_1 and compare it to $z = 1.96$. If $T_1 > 1.96$, then we reject the null hypothesis, otherwise, we do not reject it. Do this 100,000 times. Count the number of times that the null hypothesis is rejected. Check if the proportion of rejection is close to 0.025. Construct a 95% CI based on this proportion. Does this CI include 0.025?

2. Then we test a specific alternative hypothesis: Generate $n = m = 50$ observations from the following two different ordinal distributions: $F(x)$ is still the same as above. But for $G(y)$, it is now:

$P(Y = c1) = 0.01, P(Y = c2) = 0.25, P(Y = c4) = 0.30$, and $P(Y = c6) = 0.44$

Again, do the WMW test as above.

Do this 10,000 times. Find the proportion of times the null hypothesis is rejected. This is the estimated power for the WMW test for this specific alternative.

3. If the above power is much lower than 80%, the usual target for a reasonable Phase II or Phase III study, then do the simulation again, using a larger sample size for n and m. If the power is much higher than 80%, then do the simulation again, using a smaller sample size for n and m. Record these results and make a table (n,m) versus power.

4. Does the alternative hypothesis in b meet the assumption of proportional odds? Suppose we now specify an alternative hypothesis in terms of proportional odds ratios. Construct $G(y)$ accordingly first. Then carry out a simulation to find the sample size ($n = m$) for detecting OR = 2 with power = 80% at one-sided $\alpha = 0.025$. Compare the result with that from Equation 4.27.

References

Collett D. (1994). *Modelling Survival Data in Medical Research*. New York: Chapman & Hall.

CDER and CBER (US Department of Health and Human Services Food and Drug Administration Center for Drug Evaluation and Research and Center for Biologics Evaluation and Research). (2005). *Guidance for Industry: Clinical Trial Endpoints for the Approval of Cancer Drugs and Biologics*. Rockville, MD.

Fayers PM and Machin D. (2000). *Quality of Life Assessment, Analysis and Interpretation*. Chichester, UK: Wiley.

Jones B, Jarvis P, Lewis JA, and Ebbutt AF. (1996). Trials to assess equivalence: the importance of rigorous methods. *British Medical Journal* 313: 36–39.

Mann HB and Whitney DR. (1947). On a test of whether one of two random variables is stochastically larger than the other. *Annals of Mathematical Statistics* 18: 50–60.

McCullagh P. (1980). Regression models for ordinal data (with discussion). *Journal of the Royal Statistical Society,* Series B 42: 109–142.

Puntoni M, Branchi D, Argusti A, et al. (2013). A randomized, placebo-controlled, preoperative trial of allopurinol in subjects with colorectal adenoma. *Cancer Prevention Research* 6: 74–81.

Tsodikove A, Hasenclever D, and Loeffler M. (1998). Regression with bounded outcome score: evaluation of power by bootstrap and simulation in a chronic myelogenous leukaemia clinical trial. *Statistics in Medicine* 17: 1909–1922.

Walters SJ and Campbell MJ. (2005). The use of bootstrap methods for estimating sample size and analyzing health-related quality of life outcomes. *Statistics in Medicine* 24: 1075–1102.

Weisberg S. (1985). *Applied Linear Regression.* New York: Wiley.

Wilcoxon F. (1945). Individual comparisons by ranking methods. *Biometrics* 1: 80–83.

Whitehead J. (1993). Sample size calculation for ordered categorical data. *Statistics in Medicine* 12: 2257–2271.

5

Analysis of Covariance and Stratified Analysis

5.1 Principles of Data Analysis

Data analysis should tie together the study design, especially the study objective, and consequently provide appropriate interpretation of the results. For a formal data analysis, two common types of inferences are *hypothesis testing* and *estimation with confidence interval*. (Other possibilities include prediction, posterior probability, etc.; some basic Bayesian methods are introduced in Chapter 7.) The framework of hypothesis testing was used for sample size calculation in Chapter 4. Testing and estimation are both used for two aspects of the data analysis: within-group and between-group comparisons. We examine these comparisons in this chapter.

A key concept of interpretation of the results is *statistical significance* versus *clinical significance*. The former asks the question, "To what extent is the observed difference attributable to random variation?" The latter asks, "Is the observed difference clinically meaningful in magnitude?" Statistical significance is assessed by probability theory. Clinical significance is judgmental and based on consensus or expert opinion by the clinical community.

For statistical significance, the phrase "to what extent..." is often measured by the tail probability under the null hypothesis of "no difference." This tail probability is termed *p-value*. For assisting a proper interpretation of the result versus clinical significance, we often provide a 90% or 95% confidence interval with the point estimate of the treatment effect in addition to the p-value.

As we have mentioned when discussing sample size calculation, the methods of data analysis depend on the type of the outcome variable (*endpoint*); in a regression context, the outcome variable is also called the response or dependent variable:

- Continuous response—for example, blood pressure, serum cholesterol level, bone mineral density, weight, and so on. Analyses are often performed using Analysis of Variance (ANOVA) or Analysis

of Covariance (ANCOVA) on change from baseline, percent change
from baseline, or the posttreatment outcomes adjusted by the
baseline.

- Categorical—binary and ordered categorical response. For a binary
response, analyses are often performed using logistic regression with
covariates. The same is true for an ordinal categorical response using
cumulative logit models. When treatment group is the only covariate and sample size is not large, Fisher's exact test is often used for a
2×2 table. When other prognostic covariates are involved and are also
categorical, stratified analyses are performed. The Cochran–Mantel–
Haenszel test (Cochran 1954, 1957; Mantel and Haenszel 1959; Mantel
1963) is a popular stratified method to combine summary statistics
from each strata formed by the categorical prognostic variable.

- Survival response (time to event) with censoring—This endpoint
is in between binary and continuous. Cox regression assuming
proportional hazard rates and the stratified log-rank test are often
used.

We have seen some ANOVA and ANCOVA models and their roles in
previous chapters when discussing the crossover design, baseline comparability, and sample size calculations. In this chapter, we further study
ANCOVA and stratified analysis as commonly used tools for data analysis
in clinical trials to adjust for prognostic factors (covariates). We also use a
simple form of ANCOVA (a continuous response and a continuous covariate
along with treatment group) and stratified analysis (a binary response and a
binary covariate besides treatment group) to tie analysis together with some
of the key design methods such as stratification and randomization covered
in previous chapters.

In clinical trials, there could be many covariates collected, many possibly
correlated with each other. To avoid ambiguity caused by having many
possibilities of different covariates and their interactions in the data analysis,
which could lead to the problem of multiplicity and/or multicolinearity for
inference, it is good practice to prespecify a set of prognostic covariates
in the statistical analysis plan before the study is unmasked for treatment
comparisons.

5.2 Continuous Response—ANOVA and ANCOVA

An ANCOVA model contains the continuous outcome as the response
variable, and the covariates often include the baseline value of the outcome variable and other continuous or categorical variables in addition to

the treatment group. The subject's age at baseline is often a meaningful covariate to consider, because in many situations it is correlated with the subject's disease status. It can be treated as a continuous variable or be grouped on certain ranges and become a categorical variable. Therefore, ANCOVA is a method that combines ANOVA and linear regression analysis, and all of these methods are in the larger class called the general linear model (GLM). The basic idea of ANCOVA can be illustrated as follows with Figure 5.1.

Figure 5.1a shows that the observed difference in response between-treatment groups can be a result of an imbalance of a prognostic factor (covariate) or combination of factors. In this case, the treatment effect is said to be confounded with the prognostic factor(s). Hence, randomization is very important to minimize this possibility. However, imbalance can still occur by chance with randomization, especially for trials with a small sample size.

Figure 5.1b shows that even when balance is reached in the prognostic factor, the two treatment groups may still have different relationships,

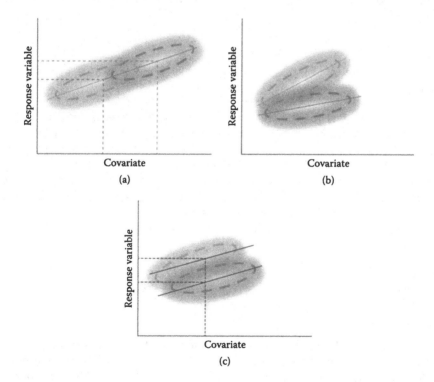

FIGURE 5.1
(a) Two treatment groups are not comparable because of differences in the covariate. (b) Two treatment groups have different correlations between response and covariate. (c) Two treatment groups are approximately comparable and have similar correlations between response and covariate.

expressed by the slopes, between the response and the prognostic factor. Treatment differences can vary at different levels of the prognostic factor. Treatment effect is shown by the difference in the slopes/correlations.

Figure 5.1c shows that there is a little imbalance (which can and often does occur even with randomization) and a little heterogeneity in slopes. We could use a common slope model to ease the analysis and interpretation. When using a common slope derived from the pooled data, the treatment difference is then considered to be constant within the range of the prognostic factor, and it simplifies the interpretation of the treatment comparison. This is the essence of ANCOVA.

In Sections 5.2.1–5.2.3, we use SAS procedures to conduct an ANCOVA step by step.

5.2.1 Test for Equal Slopes

Denote the treatment group by T, the baseline prognostic factor by X, and the outcome variable by Y. The SAS procedure for assessing equality of slopes is

```
PROC GLM;
   Class T;
   Model Y = T X T*X;
Run;
```

The ANOVA test for the treatment group by covariate interaction, T*X, indicates whether the slopes are the same across treatment groups or not. If the interaction is significant (say, at 5% level), we need to interpret the ANCOVA with caution, because this means that the treatment effects vary at different levels of the prognostic factor. In this case, we can say that the treatment effect is shown to affect the relationship, expressed by the slope, between the outcome Y and the prognostic factor X.

When the interaction is not significant, we then omit it from the MODEL statement:

```
PROC GLM;
   Class T;
   Model Y = T X;
Run;
```

In SAS, the order of the effect in the MODEL statement is important for the Type I SS (sum of squares), where the latter effect will sequentially be adjusted for the preceding effect, whereas for the Type III SS, the order is irrelevant, that is, all the effects will be adjusted for each other. In this case, it is more sensible that the treatment effect, T, is adjusted for the covariate, X. Hence, in writing T before X as seen in the MODEL statement above, the Type III SS should be used instead of the Type I SS.

When the slope is the same, the treatment comparison is adjusted for the baseline prognostic factor at any level, because the comparison will be the same regardless of the prognostic level. A meaningful choice for comparison would be at the mean level of the pooled baseline prognostic factor across the treatment groups.

When the interaction term is on the borderline of significance, we may still force a common slope (equivalent to combining the groups and fitting one regression line) to ease the interpretation of ANCOVA.

In summary, for ANCOVA, the following steps should be followed:

1. For a single factor, always make a scatter plot with a linear regression fitted for each treatment group.

2. Test the hypothesis of equal slopes.

3. If the hypothesis of equal slopes is not rejected, use a common slope ANCOVA model (i.e., a model without the interaction term) to compare the treatment difference.

4. If the slopes are shown to be significantly unequal, stop the ANCOVA. The slopes themselves express the treatment effects.

Note that the baseline measurement of the outcome variable is always considered an important prognostic factor to control by stratification and randomization methods in the study design and by the regression method in ANCOVA. We should also pay attention to the interpretation of the SAS outputs, as discussed in Section 5.2.2.

5.2.2 ANCOVA Model with a Common Slope

Let y_{ij} be the posttreatment outcome, x_{ij} be the baseline measure, and $d_{ij} = y_{ij} - x_{ij}$ be the change, for the jth patient in the ith treatment group; $i = 1, 2,$ and $j = 1, \ldots, n_i$. The ANCOVA mean model is expressed by

$$
\begin{aligned}
E(y_{ij} \mid x_{ij}) &= \mu + \tau_i + \beta(x_{ij} - \bar{x}..) \\
&= \alpha_i + \beta(x_{ij} - \bar{x}..) \\
&= \beta_0 + \tau_i + \beta x_{ij}
\end{aligned}
\tag{5.1}
$$

The term μ (or $\beta_0 = \mu - \beta\bar{X}..$) is the grand mean, τ_i (or $\alpha_i = \mu + \tau_i$) represents the effect due to treatment i, and β reflects the common linear relationship between Y and X, which is independent of the treatment group. The above expressions are equivalent, and both are presented here to make some interpretation easier in different occasions. For example, as we previously mentioned, even though the between-treatment comparison in this ANCOVA model with a common slope is the same regardless of the level of X, the first or second line of Equation 5.1 makes it clear that the comparison at the pooled average value of X (= $\bar{X}..$) is often more meaningful than at $X = 0$.

By the method of least squares (LS), we obtain the least squares estimates of the parameters:

$$\hat{\mu} = \bar{y}..$$

$$\hat{\alpha}_i = \bar{y}_i. - \hat{\beta}(\bar{x}_i. - \bar{x}..)$$

$$\hat{\beta} = \frac{\displaystyle\sum_{i=1}^{2}\sum_{j=1}^{n_i}(y_{ij} - \bar{y}..)(x_{ij} - \bar{x}..)}{\displaystyle\sum_{i=1}^{2}\sum_{j=1}^{n_i}(x_{ij} - \bar{x}..)^2}$$

$$= \frac{\displaystyle\sum_{i=1}^{2}\sum_{j=1}^{n_i}y_{ij}x_{ij} - \sum_{i=1}^{2}n_i\bar{y}_i.\bar{x}_i.}{\displaystyle\sum_{i=1}^{2}\sum_{j=1}^{n_i}x_{ij}^2 - \sum_{i=1}^{2}n_i\bar{x}_i^2.}$$

(5.2)

(At this point, if you feel that your memory of linear regression analysis is rusty, you should review this topic immediately; see Weisberg [1985].) The numerator of $\hat{\beta}$ is sometimes denoted as SS_{YX} and the denominator as SS_{XX}. Hence, in brief, $\hat{\beta} = SS_{YX}/SS_{XX}$.

In Equation 5.2, $\bar{y}_i.$ is the raw (unadjusted) mean of treatment group i, $\hat{\alpha}_i$ is the adjusted mean (LS mean) of the treatment group i, adjusted for the baseline covariate X. The amount of adjustment depends on the product of two factors: correlation of x with y (expressed by $\hat{\beta}$), and how far the group mean is away from the overall mean (i.e., degree of baseline imbalance). This is enlightening. In Chapter 2, Section 2.6, we discussed the concept of *baseline comparability*. First, using the p-value to indicate baseline comparability, as is sometimes seen in medical publications, is not as meaningful as this amount of LS mean adjustment. If we are sure that the randomization has been carried out properly, then the p-value just reflects the type I error rate. A small and statistically insignificant baseline difference (which is a type I error) of a highly correlated prognostic factor may still induce a greater adjustment than a large difference of a baseline characteristic that has very weak correlation with the outcome endpoint. Second, the design methods of stratification (for categorical covariates) and randomization can enhance the chance of baseline balance, and the method of blinding can protect the assessment bias so that the correlation between the outcome and baseline covariate would be independent of the treatment group (thus implying a common slope).

5.2.3 ANCOVA Using SAS

In addition to the mean model in Equation 5.1, the ANCOVA model also has an additive error term. When the error term is normally distributed, the LS estimators (Equation 5.2) are also the maximum likelihood estimators (MLEs). We can then perform statistical tests and confidence interval estimations. Note that testing the adjusted mean within an individual group i, $\alpha_i = 0$, by itself is not meaningful. Testing between groups, $\alpha_1 = \alpha_2$, is meaningful, by examining

$$\hat{\alpha}_1 = \bar{y}_1 . - \hat{\beta}\left(\bar{x}_1 . - \bar{x}..\right) \qquad \hat{\alpha}_2 = \bar{y}_2 . - \hat{\beta}\left(\bar{x}_2 . - \bar{x}..\right)$$

$$\hat{\alpha}_1 - \hat{\alpha}_2 = \left(\bar{y}_1 . - \bar{y}_2 .\right) - \hat{\beta}\left(\bar{x}_1 . - \bar{x}_2 .\right) \tag{5.3}$$

The adjustment for the baseline mean difference is clearly shown in Equation 5.3 here. If the randomization is fair, then $\bar{x}_1 . - \bar{x}_2 . \approx 0$, and the adjustment is nearly negligible. Hence, in the context of a properly randomized trial, especially for a randomized trial with a large sample size, the primary purpose of ANCOVA is studying covariates, not adjusting for bias. The study of covariates is a way to understand the disease and treatment mechanisms and to discover relationships that may help the investigator plan future research. Including covariates could also reduce the variance when comparing treatment effects. We discuss this point in Section 5.3.

Instead of y_{ij}, if we use d_{ij} (which is change from baseline, i.e., $d_{ij} = y_{ij} - x_{ij}$) in the ANCOVA model, what would be the slope (in relation to the above β)? Is it still meaningful to test this new slope $= 0$? Will the treatment comparison be the same as using y_{ij}? The following examines these questions.

The regression slope of the change, d, on baseline, X, is denoted by $\tilde{\beta}$. Then

$$\tilde{\beta} = \rho_{dx}\frac{\sigma_d}{\sigma_x} = \frac{\sigma_{dx}}{\sigma_d\sigma_x}\frac{\sigma_d}{\sigma_x} = \frac{\text{cov}(y-x,x)}{\sqrt{\text{var}(x)}\sqrt{\text{var}(x)}} = \frac{\text{cov}(y,x)-\text{var}(x)}{\text{var}(x)} = \beta - 1$$

Therefore, testing $\tilde{\beta} = 0$ is equivalent to testing $\beta = 1$, which is generally not meaningful, unless $\sigma_y = \sigma_x$. When $\sigma_y = \sigma_x$, $\beta = \rho$. Then, testing $\tilde{\beta} = 0$ is equivalent to testing a perfect correlation $\rho = 1$.

Now, let us look at the treatment group comparison. With obvious notation of the estimates, the LS mean of the group i is

$$\tilde{\alpha}_i = \bar{d}_i . - \hat{\beta}\left(\bar{x}_i . - \bar{x}..\right)$$

$$= \bar{d}_i . - \left(\hat{\beta} - 1\right)\left(\bar{x}_i . - \bar{x}..\right)$$

$$= \left(\bar{y}_i . - \bar{x}_i .\right) - \hat{\beta}\left(\bar{x}_i . - \bar{x}..\right) + \left(\bar{x}_i . - \bar{x}..\right)$$

$$= \bar{y}_i . - \hat{\beta}\left(\bar{x}_i . - \bar{x}..\right) - \bar{x}..$$

$$= \hat{\alpha}_i - \bar{x}..$$

Therefore, the LS mean based on y and that based on d only differ by a constant, that is, the overall average of x. The between-group comparison is the same whether using y or d. It is interesting to see from the equation

$$\tilde{\alpha}_i = \bar{d}_{i.} - \hat{\beta}\left(\bar{x}_{i.} - \bar{x}_{..}\right) \tag{5.4}$$

that testing the individual $\alpha_i = 0$ using difference, d_{ij}, is now meaningful because in this case it is now the *within-group* change from baseline, adjusted for the *regression towards the mean effect* (the second term of Equation 5.4). Note that, in contrast, the pre-post *paired t-test* only uses the first term of Equation 5.4, $\bar{d}_{i.}$, without accounting for any change attributable to regression to the mean. When the regression to the mean effect is large, we prefer Equation 5.4 for within-group change over the pre-post paired t-test.

5.3 Variance Reduction by Covariates

Following the mean model (Equation 5.1) with the error term being normally distributed with mean 0 and conditional variance var$(Y|X) = \sigma_{y|x}^2$, we can compare the unadjusted estimator of the treatment effect with the adjusted estimator in Equation 5.3. Denote the marginal variance of Y as var$(Y) = \sigma_y^2$ and assume a sample size n per group.

If the model in Equation 5.1 is correct, the unadjusted estimator of the treatment effect is $\left(\bar{y}_{1.} - \bar{y}_{2.}\right)$.

$$E\left(\bar{y}_{1.} - \bar{y}_{2.}\right) = \left(\tau_1 - \tau_2\right) + \beta\left(\bar{x}_{1.} - \bar{x}_{2.}\right)$$

This then gives a bias of $\beta\left(\bar{x}_{1.} - \bar{x}_{2.}\right)$ in estimating $\tau_1 - \tau_2$. The variance of $\left(\bar{y}_{1.} - \bar{y}_{2.}\right) = 2\sigma_y^2/n$. The mean squared error of the unadjusted estimator is therefore

$$\beta^2\left(\bar{X}_{1.} - \bar{X}_{2.}\right)^2 + 2\sigma_y^2/n \tag{5.5}$$

The adjusted estimator of the treatment effect is $\hat{\alpha}_1 - \hat{\alpha}_2 = \left(\bar{y}_1 - \bar{y}_2\right) - \hat{\beta}\left(\bar{x}_{1.} - \bar{x}_{2.}\right)$.

Because $\hat{\beta}$ is an unbiased estimator of β, $E(\hat{\alpha}_1 - \hat{\alpha}_2) = \tau_1 - \tau_2$. The variance of $\hat{\alpha}_1 - \hat{\alpha}_2$ involves the variance of $\hat{\beta}$, or more precisely, the conditional variance of $\hat{\beta}$, given X:

$$\text{Var}(\hat{\beta}|X) = \sigma_{y|x}^2/\text{SS}_{xx}.$$

Hence,

$$\text{Var}(\hat{\alpha}_1 - \hat{\alpha}_2 \mid X) = \sigma_{y|x}^2 \left[\frac{2}{n} + \frac{\left(\bar{x}_{1.} - \bar{x}_{2.}\right)}{SS_{XX}} \right] \tag{5.6}$$

Because $\hat{\alpha}_1 - \hat{\alpha}_2$ is unbiased, Equation 5.6 is also the mean squared error.

When we compare Equations 5.5 and 5.6, the desirability of adjusting the covariate for the given data relies on the unknown factors of $\sigma_{y|x}^2$, σ_y^2, and β. In practice, we can replace them with the corresponding estimates from the data. If the mean squared error (Equation 5.5) is smaller, then we use the unadjusted estimator; otherwise, we use the adjusted estimator. Some simulation studies carried out by Abeyasekera (1984) show that this strategy is better than the "always adjust" or the "always do not adjust" rules in most situations when the correlation between the response variable and the covariate is at least modest (above 0.15). This procedure is easy to do when there are only two treatment groups and only one covariate to consider. For more than one covariate and more than two treatment groups, it is more difficult to carry out.

5.4 Stratified Analysis

For a binary or ordered categorical response and some continuous and categorical covariates, logistic and cumulative logistic regression models are often used to analyze treatment effects adjusted for the covariates. Because logistic regression involves an iterative method to obtain the maximum likelihood estimates of the regression coefficient (e.g., McCullagh and Nelder 1989), it is not so obvious to perceive the impact of the distribution of the covariate as in the continuous response case by ANCOVA. However, we can make the point by studying a simple case of comparing two treatment groups ($T = A, B$) with respect to a binary response ($R = 1, 0$), stratified by a binary covariate ($X = $ "+", "−"). This stratified analysis is shown in Table 5.1.

In Table 5.1(A), the patient allocation distribution panel indicates that $P(T = A) = P(T = B) = 1/2$, meaning an even allocation between-treatment groups. $P(T = A, X = $ "+"$) = \pi_A$ and $P(T = B, X = $ "+"$) = \pi_B$ implies that $P(X = $ "+"$) = \pi_A + \pi_B$ and $P(X = $ "−"$) = 1 - \pi_A - \pi_B$. For a stratified randomization, $P(T = A \mid X = $ "+"$) = \pi_A/(\pi_A + \pi_B) = P(T = B \mid X = $ "+"$) = \pi_B/(\pi_A + \pi_B)$ if and only if $\pi_A = \pi_B$.

TABLE 5.1

Stratified Analysis

	Treatment Group (T)	
	A	B
(A) Allocation Distribution		
Factor (X) "+"	π_A	π_B
"−"	$\frac{1}{2} - \pi_A$	$\frac{1}{2} - \pi_B$
Total	$\frac{1}{2}$	$\frac{1}{2}$
(B) Response Rate		
Factor (X) "+"	$\varphi\alpha$	$\varphi\beta$
"−"	α	β
Ratio	φ	φ

The "Response Rate" panel, Table 5.1(B), indicates that

$$P(R = 1|T = A, X = \text{"−"}) = \alpha, P(R = 1|T = A, X = \text{"+"}) = \varphi\alpha,$$

$$P(R = 1|T = B, X = \text{"−"}) = \beta, P(R = 1|T = B, X = \text{"+"}) = \varphi\beta.$$

Hence,

$$P(R = 1|T = A, X = \text{"+"})/P(R = 1|T = A, X = \text{"−"})$$

$$= P(R = 1|T = B, X = \text{"+"})/P(R = 1|T = B, X = \text{"−"}) = \varphi$$

The positive factor X, that is, X = "+", influences the response rate by a multiplier of φ verses the negative factor X, that is, X = "−", independent of the treatment group. This is similar to the parallel slopes in the ANCOVA model.

From Table 5.1, we can calculate the expected response rate for each treatment group combining the strata of X = "+" and X = "−" as follows:

$$P_A = P(R = 1|T = A) = \frac{P(R = 1, T = A)}{P(T = A)} = 2[P(R = 1, T = A, X = \text{"+"})$$

$$+ P(R = 1, T = A, X = \text{"−"})]$$

$$= 2[P(R = 1|T = A, X = \text{"+"}) P(T = A, X = \text{"+"}) + P(R = 1|T = A, X = \text{"−"})$$
$$P(T = A, X = \text{"−"})]$$

$$= 2[(\varphi\alpha)\,\pi_A + \alpha(1/2 - \pi_A)]$$

$$= \alpha\,[1 + 2\pi_A(\varphi - 1)] \tag{5.7}$$

Similarly,

$$P_B = P(R = 1\,|\,T = B) = \frac{P(R = 1,\,T = B)}{P(T = B)}$$

$$= 2[(\varphi\beta)\,\pi_B + \beta(1/2 - \pi_B)]$$

$$= \beta\,[1 + 2\pi_B(\varphi - 1)] \tag{5.8}$$

To see how the treatment comparison with balanced factor X, when $\pi_A = \pi_B = \pi$, relates to that with imbalanced case, we let $\pi_A = \pi_B = \pi$ in Equations 5.7 and 5.8 and obtain, correspondingly

$$P_A^* = \alpha\left[1 + 2\pi(\varphi - 1)\right]$$

$$= P_A \frac{\left[1 + 2\pi(\varphi - 1)\right]}{\left[1 + 2\pi_A(\varphi - 1)\right]} \tag{5.9}$$

$$P_B^* = \beta\left[1 + 2\pi(\varphi - 1)\right]$$

$$= P_B \frac{\left[1 + 2\pi(\varphi - 1)\right]}{\left[1 + 2\pi_B(\varphi - 1)\right]} \tag{5.10}$$

Because the effect of X on R is expressed in term of the multiplier φ, we also examine the impact of the distribution of X in terms of ratio of response rates as follows

$$\frac{P_A}{P_B} = \frac{\alpha}{\beta}\frac{\left[1 + 2\pi_A(\varphi - 1)\right]}{\left[1 + 2\pi_B(\varphi - 1)\right]} = \frac{P_A^*}{P_B^*}\frac{\left[1 + 2\pi_A(\varphi - 1)\right]}{\left[1 + 2\pi_B(\varphi - 1)\right]} \tag{5.11}$$

The imbalance in factor X changed the ratio of response rates by a factor of $\dfrac{\left[1 + 2\pi_A(\varphi - 1)\right]}{\left[1 + 2\pi_B(\varphi - 1)\right]}$, which not only involves the distribution of X in treatment groups (π_A and π_B) but also φ, which is the effect of factor X on the response. This is an adjustment that corresponds to the additive adjustment $\beta(x_{ij} - \bar{x}..)$ in Equation 5.1 for ANCOVA.

Appendix 5.1: Weekly Average Pain Score Data

Obs	WK_0	WK_7	Age	Sex	SubjID	TRT
1	6.8571	4.5714	62	M	30007	Control
2	4.8571	2.8571	64	M	30009	Control
3	5.8571	7.0000	48	M	40003	Control
4	7.7143	5.5714	58	M	60002	Control
5	6.6000	2.0000	59	F	60007	Control
6	5.7143	6.5714	65	F	70004	Control
7	7.5714	2.2857	58	M	70012	Control
8	2.8333	0.5714	67	F	70023	Control
9	8.8571	8.7143	68	M	70037	Control
10	6.0000	1.4000	40	M	90015	Control
11	6.2857	6.0000	56	M	90025	Control
12	8.7143	7.0000	67	M	90031	Control
13	6.1429	6.1429	50	F	110001	Control
14	8.2857	8.5714	67	F	110004	Control
15	9.8000	7.8571	63	F	140014	Control
16	7.1429	5.1429	62	M	170008	Control
17	7.2857	3.8571	69	M	190004	Control
18	4.8571	2.0000	73	M	190010	Control
19	7.0000	7.0000	71	F	190015	Control
20	6.0000	1.0000	65	F	190025	Control
21	7.5714	4.8571	70	F	190036	Control
22	4.4286	2.2857	73	F	190042	Control
23	9.7143	10.0000	44	F	190046	Control
24	5.0000	3.0000	52	M	190055	Control
25	7.2857	3.8333	36	F	200002	Control
26	5.2857	2.0000	51	F	210002	Control
27	9.7143	9.0000	50	M	210009	Control
28	5.4286	3.2857	55	F	210013	Control
29	9.7143	9.3333	48	F	210014	Control
30	9.7143	10.0000	55	F	230011	Control
31	7.7143	5.0000	58	M	240001	Control
32	5.8571	5.5714	60	F	240004	Control
33	8.5714	7.7143	50	F	240012	Control
34	7.7143	8.0000	75	M	240017	Control
35	7.5714	6.0000	60	F	240023	Control
36	9.5714	9.4286	73	F	280003	Control
37	6.7143	5.1429	77	M	280010	Control
38	8.0000	5.2857	75	F	280012	Control
39	8.8571	7.2857	62	F	280015	Control

Continued

Obs	WK_0	WK_7	Age	Sex	SubjID	TRT
40	10.0000	0.0000	55	F	280016	Control
41	6.2500	5.1429	52	M	60011	Active
42	8.0000	4.4286	68	M	70010	Active
43	8.4286	9.0000	67	F	70038	Active
44	7.3333	6.8571	54	M	90004	Active
45	6.2857	4.1667	60	F	90026	Active
46	8.7500	3.2857	53	F	130001	Active
47	10.0000	1.5714	57	M	140011	Active
48	7.2857	6.3333	55	F	190054	Active
49	7.0000	5.7143	65	F	190056	Active
50	4.1429	1.1429	28	F	210008	Active
51	7.83333	4.28571	52	F	220001	Active
52	4.14286	3.42857	55	F	230001	Active
53	6.85714	4.80000	63	M	230009	Active
54	7.85714	2.57143	62	F	240005	Active
55	5.28571	5.00000	64	F	290011	Active
56	8.71429	6.00000	63	F	290046	Active
57	5.85714	3.00000	58	F	310005	Active
58	7.00000	6.57143	51	M	310033	Active
59	7.16667	8.20000	54	M	330003	Active
60	7.28571	7.42857	55	F	340004	Active
61	5.16667	4.00000	72	F	360019	Active
62	7.42857	6.28571	60	F	360023	Active
63	4.20000	6.85714	75	M	360033	Active
64	6.20000	2.42857	37	F	360046	Active
65	4.14286	2.00000	61	M	480003	Active
66	7.42857	6.14286	57	F	480008	Active
67	7.28571	8.14286	61	M	520002	Active
68	6.60000	5.85714	51	M	570009	Active
69	7.00000	7.14286	56	M	580001	Active
70	6.42857	3.00000	48	F	640003	Active
71	9.00000	7.85714	59	M	670002	Active
72	5.85714	5.00000	62	M	760002	Active
73	4.71429	0.00000	73	M	760012	Active
74	6.28571	6.00000	74	M	780004	Active
75	7.00000	6.83333	56	M	780009	Active
76	6.57143	5.66667	65	M	790010	Active
77	6.14286	0.00000	50	M	790021	Active
78	6.80000	2.85714	69	M	800003	Active
79	5.28571	5.42857	68	F	800005	Active
80	8.28571	7.00000	54	M	800014	Active
81	7.00000	1.14286	78	M	820007	Active

Homework 5.1

Appendix 5.1 lists a data set from a randomized clinical trial to evaluate treatment effect on weekly average pain score (WAPS). There are two treatment groups, Control and Active, and two measures of the WAPS, at baseline (WK_0) and Week 7 (WK_7). Patients' age and sex are also included in the list.

1. Use the WAPS at Week 7 as the response variable and at baseline as the covariate. Carry out the ANCOVA. Is the parallel slope assumption satisfied? Test the treatment effect adjusted for the covariate. Obtain the adjusted means and associated 95% CI for each treatment group.

2. Create a variable, Change in WAPS, and use it as the response variable. Include baseline WAPS, age, and sex as the covariates to carry out ANCOVA. Report the results and give your conclusions.

Homework 5.2

Stratified Analysis (Altman 1985)
1. Following the notation in Section 5.4, suppose that we have a well-balanced design by stratified randomization and obtained the following result (Table 5.2):
   a. In terms of the notation in Table 5.1, what value is φ?
   b. Test the overall treatment effect first by the combined results (100/200 vs. 80/200), then by the Cochran–Mantel–Haenszel (CMH) test. Compare and comment. (You may need to create two 2 × 2 tables to carry out the CMH test or may need to use the PROC FREQ options in SAS.)

TABLE 5.2

Homework 5.2.1: Stratified Analysis

		Treatment Group (T)			Response Rate A vs. B	
		A	**B**	**Total**		
Factor (X)	"+"	40/50	32/50	72/100	80%	64%
	"–"	60/150	48/150	108/300	40%	32%
Total		100/200	80/200	180/400	50%	40%

Source: Altman, D. G., *The Statistician*, 34, 125, 1985. With permission.

2. Without materially changing the response rates (A vs. B) in each stratum, suppose that there is imbalance in the distribution of factor X in treatment groups (A has more X = "+" and less "–" than B) as displayed in Table 5.3.
   a. Has φ changed?
   b. Use a chi-square test to check the distribution of X between-treatment groups. What is the p-value? What does this p-value represent?
   c. Test the overall treatment effect first by the combined results (103/200 vs. 77/200), then by the CMH Test. Compare and comment.

3. Without materially changing the response rates (A vs. B) in each stratum, suppose that there is imbalance in the distribution of factor X in treatment groups (B has more X = "+" and less "–" than A), as displayed in Table 5.4.
   a. Has φ changed?
   b. Use a chi-square test to check the distribution of X between-treatment groups. What is the p-value? What does this p-value represent?
   c. Test the overall treatment effect first by the combined results (97/200 vs. 83/200), then by the CMH test. Compare and comment.

TABLE 5.3

Homework 5.2.2: Stratified Analysis

		Treatment Group (T)			Response Rate A vs. B	
		A	B	Total		
Factor (X)	"+"	47/59	26/41	73/100	80%	63%
	"–"	56/141	51/159	107/300	40%	32%
Total		103/200	77/200	180/400	51.5%	38.5%

Source: Altman, D. G., *The Statistician*, 34, 125, 1985. With permission.

TABLE 5.4

Homework 5.2.3: Stratified Analysis

		Treatment Group (T)			Response Rate A vs. B	
		A	B	Total		
Factor (X)	"+"	33/41	38/59	71/100	80%	64%
	"–"	64/159	45/141	109/300	40%	32%
Total		97/200	83/200	180/400	48.5%	41.5%

Source: Altman, D. G., The Statistician, 34, 125, 1985. With permission.

References

Abeyasekera S. (1984). The desirability of covariance adjustments. *Journal of the Royal Statistical Society. Series C (Applied Statistics)* 33: 33–37.

Altman DG. (1985). Comparability of randomized groups. *The Statistician* 34: 125–136.

Cochran WG. (1954). Some methods for strengthening the common chi-square tests. *Biometrics* 21: 86–98.

Cochran WG. (1957). Analysis of covariance. Its nature and uses. *Biometrics* 13: 261–281.

Mantel N and Haenszel W. (1959). Statistical aspects of the analysis of data from retrospective studies. *Journal of the National Cancer Institute* 2: 719–748.

Mantel N. (1963). Chi-square tests with one-degree of freedom: extensions of the Mantel-Haenszel procedure. *Journal of the American Statistical Association* 58: 690–700.

McCullagh P and Nelder JA. (1989). *Generalized Linear Models*. London: Chapman & Hall.

Weisberg S. (1985). *Applied Linear Regression*. New York: Wiley.

6

Sequential Designs and Methods—Part I: Expected Sample Size and Two-Stage Phase II Trials in Oncology

In Chapter 4, we mainly considered the fixed sample size design, in which there is no interim analysis. As we alluded to in Chapter 1, however, clinical trials often require periodic monitoring and data analyses at interim stages, while patients are continuously enrolled. This monitoring and analysis is especially necessary for trials that involve life-threatening diseases, potentially toxic therapies, long-term follow-ups, or large sample sizes. In this chapter and in Chapter 7, we examine sequential designs and methods for clinical trials with interim stages, with an illustration using oncology trials.

As we discussed in previous chapters, all considerations for making a fixed sample size trial valid and efficient are also pertinent to sequentially designed trials (or *sequential trials* for short). In sequential trials, we need to focus special attention on control of the overall type I error rate (α) and the impact of the target study power ($1 - \beta$) with any interim analyses. We also need to carefully preserve the integrity of the trial as more issues emerge with the possibility to introduce bias, especially because the trial remains ongoing and thereby offers a chance to alter the process when results are being monitored. (For example, we would not discontinue sites with poor results.) In addition, we need to set up *decision rules* or *guidelines* for possible early termination or other modification of the study within the protocol or the *data analysis plan*, or both.

6.1 Maximum Sample Size and Expected Sample Size

When we design a sequential trial with a total sample size N, this N is actually the final projected sample size, if the trial continues to the end. As a sequential trial, the study might be terminated early, for example, in the middle of accrual, and thus this N would not be achieved. Therefore, unlike a nonsequential (fixed sample size) trial, the sample size in a sequential trial is actually not a fixed number. The designed N in the sequential trials is the possible *maximum sample size* for the study. There is also a concept of *expected sample size* in trials with a sequential design.

In order to reach the same statistical power, a sequential trial would require a larger *maximum sample size* than the corresponding fixed sample size for a nonsequential design. Hence, in order to plan a sequential trial, we should first use the sample size formula we discussed and learned in Chapter 4 and then increase this sample size number to obtain a corrected sample size for the corresponding sequential study. This increase of the maximum sample size also reflects a potential cost for conducting the extra monitoring of the study. However, the expected sample size for a sequential trial would be smaller with the chance of an early termination.

To illustrate these points, let us consider the distinctive characteristics of the Phase II cancer trials in the following section.

6.2 One-Stage versus Two-Stage Cancer Phase II Trials

6.2.1 Introduction

The main objective of a Phase II cancer trial is to determine whether a new therapy (usually a combination of agents or treatment regimens and modalities) has sufficient activity against a specific type of tumor to warrant further (Phase III) development. A major difference between cancer Phase II trials and trials involving many other diseases is that the former are usually designed as a single-arm trial without a concurrent control. Instead, historical data controls are often considered for comparison. (Extensive epidemiologic data, literature review, and meta-analysis are crucial to the interpretation of a Phase II cancer trial using historical controls.) The primary endpoint for cancer Phase II trials is usually the tumor response rate as defined clinically, based on a combination of reduction in tumor size and/or changes in biochemical markers, and more recently event-free (e.g., progression-free) survival at a fixed time point. For example, in the year 2000, an international committee standardized easily applicable criteria known as *Response Evaluation Criteria in Solid Tumors* (*RECIST*) for measuring solid tumor response using x-ray, CT, and MRI technology. *RECIST* is recommended for most NCI-sponsored trials. When a single (overall) *response rate* is calculated, *complete* and *partial responses* (CR+PR) are usually pooled together, versus *progressive disease* and *stable disease* (PD+SD). Sometimes investigators also collect data on survival, but confidence intervals are usually very wide due to the small sample size.

Hypothesis testing for a Phase II trial is usually based on response rates, because the response facilitates the decision of whether or not to proceed to a Phase III trial. The therapy would be deemed uninteresting if the true response rate (p) were no more than a certain level (p_0) and would be accepted for further investigation in larger groups of patients (i.e., Phase III studies) if the true response were greater than some target level (p_1). The level for the uninteresting response rate (p_0) would most likely be derived from the literature regarding standard therapy. The target level of response rate (i.e., the alternative hypothesis, p_1) is usually set based on the investigator's expectation of the new therapy to be interesting for further study, but it should also be realistic and based on earlier or preclinical data. Typically, for ethical and practical considerations, a two- or three-stage design is used for these Phase II trials, so that an ineffective treatment can be dismissed early at the end of the first stage. In the early 1960s, when anticancer agents showed low activity, Gehan's (1961) two-stage design was used widely, in which p_0 was set to be zero. Later, Simon (1989) generalized p_0 and introduced *optimal* and *minimax designs*. The optimal design minimizes the expected sample size under the null hypothesis and the minimax design minimizes the maximum of the total sample size.

6.2.2 Review of the Binomial Distribution and Sample Size Estimation for a One-Sample Case Using R Functions

Recall that the *binomial distribution table* in a fundamental statistics textbook was used when we applied the *sign test* in Homework 3.2 (Chapter 3) for analyzing paired data from a crossover study. We now use the functions in the R package to implement the calculations. First, the *binomial density function* is

$$b(x;n,p) = \binom{n}{x} p^x (1-p)^{n-x}$$

The probability of having x responses out of n patients (sample size) when the chance of response is p (prob) can be obtained by using the R function:

```
dbinom(x, size, prob)
```

Second, the *binomial cumulative probability* is

$$B(r;n,p) = \sum_{x=0}^{r} b(x;n,p)$$

The probability of having at most r responses ($\leq r$) out of n patients when the chance of response is p can be obtained by using the R function:

```
pbinom(x, size, prob)
```

The hypotheses in a single-arm trial are H_0: $p = p_0$ and H_A: $p = p_1$, and the associated sample size with the type I (α) and type II ($1 - \beta$) errors is

$$n = \frac{\left[z_{\alpha/2} \sqrt{p_0(1-p_0)} + z_\beta \sqrt{p_1(1-p_1)} \right]^2}{(p_1 - p_0)^2} \tag{6.1}$$

The above notation is best illustrated with an example. The response rate for the standard therapy for refractory Hodgkin's disease is 50% (p_0). A new experimental combination therapy is to be tested, and the investigator expects a response rate of 80% (p_1) for the new therapy. Assume a fixed sample size design is conducted with n = 10 patients. Let X be the number of responses in the 10 patients. Suppose we design the trial with the following decision rule: Dismiss the drug if X ≤ 7 (i.e., accept H_0). Claim the drug is worthy of further study if X ≥ 8. We need to understand the *operating characteristics* of this rule.

The type I error rate is α = Pr(X ≥ 8 | n = 10, p = p_0 = 0.5) = 1 – Pr(X ≤ 7 | n = 10, p = p_0 = 0.5). With R we obtain

```
1-pbinom(7,10,p = 0.5)
[1] 0.0546875
```

The type II error rate is β = Pr(X ≤ 7 | n = 10, p = p_1 = 0.8). The power is 1 – β = 1 – Pr(X ≤ 7 | n = 10, p = p_1 = 0.8). For power, we obtain from R

```
1-pbinom(7,10,p = 0.8)
[1] 0.6777995
```

Investigators often monitor cancer trials as they are ongoing. For example, in the above trial, suppose that there are only three responses after the first five patients. An interesting question then is, should the trial be continued? Before we tackle this question in the next section, we should bear in mind that one should not do an unplanned sequential monitoring of a fixed sample size trial. If that were done, then the error rates would no longer be controlled at the nominal level. When it is desirable to have an interim analysis, then the study team should consider a two-stage design in the protocol.

6.2.3 Example of a Two-Stage Design

Suppose we alter the above example a little bit as follows.

- Stage I: Enter n_1 = 5 patients. If X_1 ≤ 3 responses are observed, then stop the study and dismiss the drug. Otherwise, continue to the next stage.
- Stage II: Enter another n_2 = 5 patients. Out of the total n = $n_1 + n_2$ = 10, if X = $X_1 + X_2$ ≥ 8 responses are observed, then reject the null hypothesis and claim the drug is worthy of further study.

In other words, we now add an interim stage to monitor the study. Note that the first stage only stops the trial for futility (i.e., when the response rate is poor). This approach is used to save resources, as well as to avoid giving additional patients an ineffective therapy. This approach does not stop the trial at the first stage when the response *appears* to be effective, because this is only a small Phase II study. When we successfully pass the interim target level, we continue the trial to its designed end. At the end of the study, we can either dismiss the drug from further (Phase III) testing (i.e., accept the null hypothesis) or permit the drug to be tested in further (Phase III) trials (i.e., reject the null hypothesis).

Given the above design configuration ($n_1 = 5$, $r_1 = 3$, $n = 10$, $r = 7$), we ask: What are the *operating characteristics* of this two-stage sequential design? Specifically, we calculate the type I error and type II error rates, the probability of early termination (PET), and the expected sample size.

The following basic rule of probability will be applied repeatedly in a sequential design:

$$\Pr(A \text{ and } B) = \Pr(B|A)P(A) = \sum_a \Pr(B|A = a)\Pr(A = a) \qquad (6.2)$$

- First, the type I error rate $\alpha = \Pr(\text{reject } H_0 | H_0) = P(\text{pass the first stage,}$ and then observe at least $r = 8$ responses out of $n = 10$ patients $|$ $p = 0.5$); while passing the first stage we need $X_1 \geq 4$ responses out of $n_1 = 5$. Therefore,

  $\alpha = \Pr(\text{get } X \geq 8 \text{ responses out of } n = 10 \text{ patients} | \text{already have } 4$ responses from $n_1 = 5$ patients, $p = 0.5$) $\times \Pr(4 \text{ responses from } n_1 = 5,$ $p = 0.5$) $+ \Pr(\text{get } X \geq 8 \text{ responses out of } n = 10 \text{ patients} | 5 \text{ responses}$ from $n_1 = 5$, $p = 0.5$) $\times \Pr(5 \text{ responses from } n_1 = 5, p = 0.5)$

  $= \Pr(\text{get } X_2 \geq 4 \text{ responses out of } n_2 = 10 - n_1 = 5, p = 0.5) \times 0.15625 +$ $\Pr(\text{get } X_2 \geq 3 \text{ responses out of } n_2 = 5, p = 0.5) \times 0.03125 = 0.1875 \times$ $0.15625 + 0.5 \times 0.03125 = 0.0449.$

  The above calculation can be carried out in R:

  ```
  > (1-pbinom(3,5,0.5))*dbinom(4,5,0.5) + (1-pbinom
     (2,5,0.5))*dbinom(5,5,0.5)
  [1] 0.04492188
  ```

- Next, the power is obtained similarly by

  $1 - \beta = \Pr(\text{reject } H_0 | H_A) = \Pr(\text{pass the first stage, then observe at}$ least $r = 8$ responses out of $n = 10$ patients $| p = 0.8$)

  With R,

  ```
  > (1-pbinom(3,5,0.8))*dbinom(4,5,0.8) + (1-pbinom
     (2,5,0.8))*dbinom(5,5,0.8)
  [1] 0.6106907
  ```

- Third, the PET. Early termination occurs when we observe $X_1 \leq 3$ responses out of $n_1 = 5$ patients at the first stage. There are actually two PETs to consider.

PET under H_0: $\Pr(X_1 \leq 3; n_1 = 5, p = 0.5)$

```
>pbinom(3,5,0.5)
[1] 0.8125
```

PET under H_A: $\Pr(X_1 \leq 3; n_1 = 5, p = 0.8)$

```
>pbinom(3,5,0.8)
[1] 0.26272
```

Note that PET under H_0 is much greater than PET under H_A. This fact is intuitive because, if the experimental therapy is not working as well as expected (p = 0.5 only), we would like to terminate the trial early.

- *Expected sample size.* The expected sample size is a weighted average of sample sizes of the stages. We also calculate two expected sample sizes following the two PETs. In general,

$$E(N) = \sum_k k \times p(N = k) \tag{6.3}$$

In our situation, the total sample size $N = n_1 = 5$ if the trial stops after stage 1, or $N = 10$ if it does not stop after Stage 1. We already calculated PET = 0.8125 under H_0 and PET = 0.2627 if H_A is true. Hence,

$$E(N|H_0) = 5 \times 0.8125 + 10(1 - 0.8125) = 5.94$$

$$E(N|H_A) = 5 \times 0.2627 + 10(1 - 0.2627) = 8.69$$

Note that, if the therapy does not work well (p = 0.5), we would expect the study to terminate earlier, hence fewer patients are tested compared to when it works well (six versus nine). The expected sample size in both cases is less than the maximum sample size $N = 10$.

We summarize the above illustration in Table 6.1 with the following comparisons: A two-stage design requires the configuration of four parameters

TABLE 6.1

Two-Stage versus One-Stage Designs

	Two-Stage	**One-Stage**
α	0.045	0.055
$1 - \beta$	0.611	0.678
E(N)	5.94 (under H_0)	10
	8.69 (under H_A)	

Note: H_0: $p = p_0 = 0.5$, and H_A: $p = p_1 = 0.8$.

(such as $n_1 = 5, r_1 = 3, n = 10, r = 7$), as opposed to the one-stage fixed size design, where only two parameters are needed (e.g., $n = 10, r = 7$). To test the same hypotheses with the same maximum sample size ($n = 10$), we have seen that the one-stage design has a greater power (0.678) and a higher type I error rate (0.055), compared to the two-stage design (0.611 and 0.045, respectively). This is because the above two-stage design increases the chance of accepting the null hypothesis with an interim analysis for futility (i.e., increases type II error rate, hence lowers the power). The decrease in the type I error rate in the above two-stage design is because the rejection of the null hypothesis can only occur at the final stage when the interim data have passed through from the first stage. Later when we discuss a general sequential design that also allows for early rejection of the null hypothesis at the interim stages, we find an increase of the type I error rate. In addition, note that the two-stage design has a smaller expected sample size, which is a major advantage of the sequential design.

The above example also illustrates how to obtain the statistical properties of a given two-stage design with a configuration represented by (n_1, r_1, n, r). These statistical properties include α, $1-\beta$, and $E(N)$ (Homework 6.1). A natural question following this illustration is, with a given (α, β) for testing a specific H_0 (p_0) versus H_A (p_1), how do we find a design with a configuration (n_1, r_1, n, r) that indicates the maximum and interim sample sizes, decision rules, and $E(N)$? These topics are discussed in Section 6.3. Also note that one may also be interested in calculating the probability of abandoning the drug (Homework 6.2).

6.3 Simon's Two-Stage Designs

There are two kinds of designs proposed in Simon (1989): 1) optimal design and 2) minimax design. The optimal design is the one where the expected sample size under the null hypothesis is the smallest among all feasible designs. The minimax design is the one where the maximum sample size is the smallest one among all feasible designs. A design is feasible if the configuration satisfies the constraints of the type I and type II error rates. The algorithm to search and construct these two designs is described in Sections 6.3.1 and 6.3.2.

6.3.1 Optimal Design

For specified values (p_0, p_1, α, β), fix a large N (e.g., $N = 55$). All configurations with $n \leq N$ are searched. For each n_1 in the range of ($1, n-1$), we determine the integer values of (r_1, r), with r_1 in ($0, n_1$) and r in (r_1, n), so that the type I error rate is controlled at α and the type II error rate is controlled at β. (We demonstrated the calculation of α and β in the previous section.) Then from all the feasible solutions we choose the one with the smallest $E(N|p = p_0)$.

(We also demonstrated the calculation of the $E(N|p = p_0)$ in Section 6.2.) Note that $E(N|p = p_0)$ is chosen to reflect the goal of stopping early if the drug does not work (futility).

6.3.2 Minimax Design

We start with the fixed sample size n given by Equation 6.1. Recall that a sequential design requires a larger maximum sample size than the fixed size design. Thus, this n is our lower bound. If we find a solution, we stop and obtain (n_1, r_1, n, r); otherwise, we increase n to n+1 and repeat the algorithm. The algorithm of finding a solution is similar to that for the optimal design: for each n_1 in the range (1, n–1), determine the integer values of (r_1, r), with r_1 in $(0, n_1)$ and r in (r_1, n) to satisfy the constraints of type I and type II error rates (α, β). Do this until we finish with n_1 for that n. Note that, because we started from the lower bound for n and increased to the next n+1, we stop when a solution is found. Thus, this process chooses a solution that has the smallest n, the maximum sample size of the study.

6.4 Discussion

6.4.1 Software

The paper by Simon (1989) contains tables for many commonly used design configurations. Computer programs are also available for calculating Simon's two-stage designs. For example, a website at the National Cancer Institute[*] and the NCSS/PASS site[†] can be used for this purpose. In addition, many NCI designated cancer centers also have accessible computer programs on their websites, such as the Vanderbilt-Ingram Cancer Center.[‡] Another useful resource is the Clinical Trial Design Systems (CTDSystems) at the Duke Cancer Institute.[§] The CTDSystem is especially useful because it also provides a graphical display of the optimal and minimax designs (Homework 6.3).

6.4.2 P-value

Following the notation in Section 6.2.3, we give the p-value for a study with Simon's 2-stage design. (Note: The p-value is the probability of getting the

---

[*] NCI website: http://linus.nci.nih.gov/brb/samplesize/otsd.html

[†] NCSS/PASS website: http://www.ncss.com/

[‡] Vanderbilt-Ingram Cancer Center (2007). Available at http://www.vicc.org/biostatistics/ts/twostage.php

[§] Duke Cancer Institute. "Clinical Trial Design Systems," available at http://www.dukecancer-institute.org/research/shared-resources/biostatistics/clinical-trial-design-systems/

same or a more extreme result as the observed value in the direction of the alternative under the null hypothesis.)

For a case in which the trial is stopped at the first stage due to futility, that is, $x_1 \leq r_1$, the p-value is given by

$$\Pr(X_1 \geq x_1 \mid n_1, p = p_0) = 1 - \Pr(X_1 \leq x_1 - 1 \mid n_1, p = p_0)$$

$$= 1 - B(x_1 - 1; \mid n_1, p = p_0) \tag{6.4}$$

This can be easily obtained with the R function: $1\text{–pbinom}(x_1\text{–}1, n_1, p = p_0)$.

For a case in which $x_1 > r_1$, the trial continues to the second stage with an additional n_2 patients and x_2 responses. The p-value is calculated by

$$\Pr(X_1 > r_1, X_1 + X_2 \geq x_1 + x_2 \mid n_1, n_2, p = p_0)$$

$$= \sum_{x=r_1+1}^{\min(n_1,\, x_1+x_2-1)} \Pr(X_1 = x \mid n_1, p = p_0) \Pr(X_1 + X_2 \geq x_1 + x_2 \mid X_1 = x, n_2, p = p_0)$$

$$= \sum_{x=r_1+1}^{\min(n_1,\, x_1+x_2-1)} \Pr(X_1 = x \mid n_1, p = p_0) \Pr(X_2 \geq x_1 + x_2 - x \mid n_2, p = p_0) \tag{6.5}$$

$$= \sum_{x=r_1+1}^{\min(n_1,\, x_1+x_2-1)} b(x; n_1, p_0) \left[1 - B(x_1 + x_2 - x - 1; n_2, p_0)\right]$$

(because X_1 and X_2 are independent cohorts of patients). It is obvious that $X_1 = x \leq n_1$, and that $x_1 + x_2 - x - 1 \geq 0$, thus $x \leq x_1 + x_2 - 1$. Hence, the upper limit for x is $\min(n_1, x_1 + x_2 - 1)$ (Homework 6.4).

6.4.3 Other Issues

A common issue of concern with Simon's design is its rigid rules. In practice, trials are often interrupted for additional review of the study status or end up with deviations from the original design; either fewer patients enrolled due to accrual shortage or more patients enrolled due to over-running. Koyama and Chen (2008) discussed proper inference when deviation occurs at the second stage, including p-value adjustment, point estimate and confidence interval calculations for the response rate. Their software is available online (Homework 6.5).* Wu and Shih (2008) tackled the issue of redesign when interruption and deviation occurs.

---

* Koyama, T., Chen, H., and Gray, W. (2009). "Proper Inference from Simon's Two-Stage Designs," available at http://biostat.mc.vanderbilt.edu/wiki/Main/TwoStageInference

Homework 6.1

How does the expected sample size E(N) relate to the PET (probability of early termination) in a two-stage design with n_1 in the first stage and total $n = n_1 + n_2$ at the end of the trial? Give a precise mathematical expression.

Homework 6.2

Consider a single-arm, two-stage design for a Phase II cancer trial. We test H_0: $p = 0.5$ versus H_A: $p = 0.8$, where p is the response rate of the new compound. The two-stage design is as follows:

Stage I: Enter $n_1 = 5$ patients. If observe $X_1 \leq 3$ responses, stop the study and dismiss the drug. Otherwise, continue to the next stage.

Stage II: Enter another $n_2 = 5$ patients. Out of the total $n = n_1 + n_2 = 10$, if observe $X \geq 8$ responses, reject the null hypothesis and claim the drug is worthy of further study.

    a. Calculate the probability that this compound will be abandoned/ dismissed from further studies if the true response rate is 0.5.

    b. Calculate the probability of abandoning further studies if the true response rate is 0.8.

Homework 6.3

Read the following paper: "A Phase II Study of Sorafenib in Patients with Platinum-Pretreated, Advanced (Stage IIIb or IV) Non-Small Cell Lung Cancer with a KRAS Mutation" (Dingemans, A. M., et al., *Clinical Cancer Research*, 2013, 19(3): 743–51).

    1. What was the primary endpoint of this study?

    2. This study used Simon's two-stage optimal design. Find what the assumed parameters were for the design.

    3. Check the design decision rules given in the paper with the software given in the chapter.

    4. What would the decision rules have been if Simon's minimax design had been used instead? Discuss the merits of the optimal design versus the minimax design in this case.

5. Comment on the result of the study with regard to the primary endpoint as reported in the paper, compared with the design.

6. What would the sample size have been if a one-stage fixed sample size design were used instead, with the same hypotheses, type I error rate, and power? Compare it with the maximum sample size and expected sample size of the two-stage optimal design used by the study.

Homework 6.4

1. Write a program in R to calculate the p-value in Equation 6.5.

2. Calculate the p-value for a hypothetical scenario where $x_1 = 6$ and $x_2 = 4$ under the design ($n_1 = 7$, $r_1 = 4$, $n = 20$, $r = 13$) for testing $H_0: p = p_0 = 0.5$ versus $H_A: p = p_1 = 0.8$.

Homework 6.5

A Phase II clinical trial was conducted to determine the overall response (CR + PR) of a combination therapy with paclitaxel, 13-cis retinoic acid, and interferon alfa-2b in women with Stage IVB or recurrent cervical cancer. The response rate was expected to be greater than that of paclitaxel alone in the referenced historical studies of 18%. The combination therapy was considered clinically interesting if the response rate was greater than 30%. Simon's two-stage optimal design was applied, with type I error rate = 0.10 and power = 0.80.

1. Verify that the optimal design's solution is $(n_1, r_1, n, r) = (27, 5, 66, 15)$, and interpret this configuration.

2. It turned out that there were $x_1 = 9$ responders (CR + PR) during the first stage and the study continued to the second stage. However, because of slow accrual, the protocol was closed after only 6 additional patients were accrued. In the second stage 1/6 patients had a partial response. Use the method and software of Koyama and Chen (2008) to obtain the p-value, the median estimate, and the 90% confidence interval of the response rate (CR + PR). Comment on whether the p-value and the confidence interval give the same conclusion or not.

References

Dingemans AM, Mellema WW, Groen HJ, van Wijk A, Burgers SA, Kunst PW, Thunnissen E. (2013). A Phase II study of Sorafenib in patients with platinum-pretreated, advanced (Stage IIIb or IV) non–small cell lung cancer with a KRAS mutation. *Clinical Cancer Research* 19: 743–751.

Gehan, EA. (1961). The determination of the number of patients required in a preliminary and a follow-up of a new chemotherapeutic agent. *Journal of Chronic Disease* 13: 346–353.

Koyama T and Chen H. (2008). Proper inference from Simon's two-stage designs. *Statistics in Medicine* 27: 3145–3154.

Simon, RM. (1989). Optimal two-stage designs for Phase II clinical trials. *Controlled Clinical Trials* 10: 1–10.

Wu Y and Shih WJ. (2008). Approaches to handling data when a Phase II trial deviates from the pre-specified Simon's two-stage design. *Statistics in Medicine* 27: 6190–6208.

7

Sequential Designs and Methods—Part II: Monitoring Safety and Futility

7.1 Monitoring Safety

We started with a definition of a clinical trial in Chapter 1, which led to the immediate concern of conducting experiments with human beings. We further highlighted ethics and regulations regarding the trial participant's right to privacy, information on risk and benefit, and safety protection. In order to remain ethically compliant with these intents, we must monitor and protect the subject's safety periodically throughout the trial. When the risks of continuing the trial outweigh the potential benefits, the trial should be modified or even stopped to protect the safety of those already in the trial, as well as to prevent exposure to the risk for those who are yet to be recruited. Similarly, if early superiority (efficacy) is clearly demonstrated, modification or even early termination of the trial should be considered, because it is unethical to continue subjects on the inferior arm. Stopping or modification for efficacy is discussed in Chapter 8.

7.1.1 Adverse Events

An *adverse event* (AE) is any untoward medical occurrence in a subject participating in a clinical study who is administered a medical (investigational or noninvestigational) product. An AE may not necessarily relate causally to the treatment. An AE can therefore be any unfavorable and unintended sign (including an abnormal laboratory finding), symptom, event, or disease temporally associated with the use of the product, whether or not it is related to that product or device (EMA 1995, NCI 2009). An AE in a clinical trial is commonly classified based on the investigator's judgment on

- *relationship* to the study medication, as definitely, probably, possibly related, or not likely related.
- *severity*, as mild, moderate, or severe intensity.
- *seriousness*, as yes or no. A serious AE (SAE) is any adverse experience that (i) results in death; (ii) is life-threatening; (iii) requires inpatient

hospitalization or prolongation of existing hospitalization; (iv) results in persistent, permanent, or significant disability/incapacity; (v) is a congenital anomaly/birth defect; (vi) is a suspected transmission of any infectious agent via a medicinal product; or (v) is judged medically important for expedited reporting and/or emergent intervention to prevent one of the outcomes listed above (such as suicide attempt) (EMA 1995).

All AEs should be reported in the CRF. The accompanying information also includes the AE start date and time (to determine whether the AE is "treatment emergent"), duration, action taken, and the outcome—whether resolved, worsened, improved, or continuing on the day of the report. AEs are identified by clinical history, physical examinations, and laboratory tests. The FDA and other regulatory agencies require that all AEs, regardless of how remotely they are considered to be related, be collected and reported. An example of this might be illustrated in reporting (severe) traffic accidents following therapy, with the idea that some extremely remotely associated events might, if seen with some frequency, actually have a relationship with the treatment.

Clinical AEs are further grouped according to the body system and organ class involved (cardiac, eye, hepatobiliary, infections and infestations, gastrointestinal, musculoskeletal and connective tissue, nervous system, psychiatric, renal and urinary, respiratory, thoracic, skin, etc.).

Laboratory AEs are measured by urine and blood tests. ECG, *vital signs* (blood pressures, pulse rate, weight, height, and perhaps body temperature and respiratory rate for some lung studies), and physical examination findings are also analyzed. It is more meaningful to analyze the laboratory data and vital signs by comparing changes from baseline with regard to the *normal ranges* rather than calculating the mean or median. For multicenter trials, a central laboratory should be used to standardize the tests and normal ranges, especially for any tests that are new or not part of the standardized tests monitored by laboratory accrediting agencies such as the American College of Pathology. In data analyses, the laboratory values are classified as below, within, or above the normal ranges—sometimes twice or three times the upper or lower limits of the normal ranges (ULN and LLN respectively). For example, for drugs that may induce liver injury, Hy's Law specifies that subjects with any elevated AT (AST or ALT) of >3xULN and ALP <2xULN, associated with an increase in bilirubin ≥2xULN, should be examined with special attention (FDA 2007). So, for statisticians this can become a 3×3 pre-versus-post treatment ordinal categorical data problem, testing for symmetry versus asymmetry within each treatment group.

For data analyses, issues with multiple tests arise when many routine lab tests and clinical examinations are performed. Some prefer conservativeness for safety without any adjustment of the p-values. Some advocate for a tier system prioritizing the tests and examinations for a predefined set of AEs that are known to occur with other drugs of the same class, such as GI bleeding for NSAIDs, cardiac events for COX-II inhibitors, thrombocytopenia (low blood platelet count) for sulfa-containing antibiotics and anticonvulsants (e.g., heparin), vomiting and hair loss for certain cancer treatments, hypoglycemia for antidiabetic drugs, and so on. Special attention should be paid to this predefined set of AEs (called AEs of special interest). Routine labs and examinations are generally analyzed for exploratory purposes.

7.1.2 Monitoring SAEs Using Bayesian Methods

As discussed above, except for the prespecified treatment-class-related AEs, it is usually not appropriate to use significance tests for monitoring safety endpoints due to the issue of multiplicity. Other methods may be more suitable for answering clinical questions. In this chapter a basic Bayesian method is introduced that has been used for trials involving chemotherapy, immunotherapy, and peripheral stem cell transplantation in treating patients with *multiple myeloma*.

With high-dose chemotherapy and autologous stem cell transplantation for patients with multiple myeloma, risk of severe myelotoxicity, mucositis, life-threatening infections and early mortality are all prominent complications. Furthermore, for allogeneic transplantation following chemoimmunotherapy, early allogeneic graft failure, and severe acute graft-versus-host disease (GVHD) after treatment regimen are additional serious concerns (Eastern Cooperative Oncology Group 2001). In these scenarios, it is desirable to have a close monitoring plan as each patient is treated in the trial. This is known as *continuous monitoring* (as opposed to group sequential monitoring, discussed in the next chapter), which is only suitable for an *immediate response* type of endpoint. If a critical number of predefined serious events is reached, the study should be stopped. Otherwise, the study may continue. The question is, what is that critical number?

7.1.3 The Beta-Binomial Model

The monitoring process can be formulated as follows. The event rate associated with the tested treatment is denoted by θ. Let θ^* be a predefined threshold value (e.g., 0.15). When (x, n) is observed, where x is the number of events out of n treated patients, we calculate the *posterior probability* of the event rate exceeding the threshold: $p = \Pr(\theta > \theta^* \mid x \text{ out of } n)$. The study is stopped if p is very high, say, 80%. Otherwise, the study may continue. In a Bayesian framework, the event rate θ is regarded as a random variable with a probability distribution, not as a fixed parameter. For any given θ, 'X out of n' follows the binomial distribution, that is, $X \sim \text{binom}(n;\theta)$. Recall that in Chapter 6 we used its pdf and cdf in R:

```
dbinom(x, size, prob)
pbinom(x, size, prob, lower.tail = TRUE)
```

The fundamental *Bayes' theorem* is the following probability relationship:

$$Pr(A \mid B) = \frac{Pr(B \mid A) \, Pr(A)}{Pr(B)} \tag{7.1}$$

This rule is very useful when we want to know the *conditional or posterior probability* of A given B, but what we have is the reverse information: the conditional probability of B given A. However, we also need the *marginal probability* of A, which is the *prior* probability in the Bayesian framework. The denominator Pr(B) is a normalization constant because we are conditioning on B.

Incidentally, Bayes' theorem is also the basis for calculating information regarding diagnosis of a disease with a medical device. In such a situation, Bayes' rule expresses

Pr(true disease | observed symptom)

$$= \frac{Pr(symptom \mid disease) \, Pr(disease)}{Pr(symptom)}$$

where Pr(true disease status | observed symptom) is commonly known as the *positive predictive value* (PPV), Pr(symptom | disease) is the *sensitivity* of the diagnostic device, and Pr(disease) is the *prevalence* of the disease. These are familiar terms in a public health context.

When there are n patients being treated, we evaluate

$$Pr\left(\theta > \theta^* \mid x \text{ out of } n\right) = \int_{\theta^*}^{1} f(\theta \mid x, n) \, d\theta \tag{7.2}$$

by applying Bayes' rule to the posterior pdf

$$f(\theta \mid x, n) = f(x \mid \theta, n) \, f(\theta) / f(x \mid n) \tag{7.3}$$

The posterior pdf is viewed as a function of θ for the given data (x, n). The marginal pdf in the denominator is the normalization constant of the posterior pdf and it does not include θ. To find the posterior distribution with a *conjugate prior*, it often suffices to write

$$f(\theta \mid x, n) \propto f(x \mid \theta, n) \, f(\theta) \tag{7.4}$$

In other words, "the posterior is proportional to the product of the likelihood of the data and the prior distribution."

The beta-binomial relationship is a convenient model for binary endpoints, because the beta distribution is the conjugate prior of the binomial distribution. It works as follows. With $f(x \mid \theta, n)$ as a binomial pdf binom(x, n, θ) ∝ θ^x (1−θ)$^{n-x}$ for a given (θ,n), the corresponding conjugate distribution as a function of θ is the beta distribution with shape parameters (a, b) with pdf beta(a, b) ∝ θ^{a-1}(1−θ)$^{b-1}$. Following Equation 7.4, the posterior $f(\theta|x,n)$ ∝ θ^{a+x-1}(1−θ)$^{b+n-x-1}$ has the form of a beta distribution with parameters (a+x, b+n−x). In the context of the data (x, n), the (hyper-)parameters (a, b) for the beta distribution can be interpreted as, prior to observing the data, a being the number of events out of a+b hypothetical subjects. The *beta-binomial model* containing a beta posterior with parameters (a+x, b+n−x) indicates that, after getting the data, the number of events and subjects yields a+b+n and a+x, respectively. The choice of parameters of the prior distribution will determine how much influence the "prior knowledge" will contribute to the final (posterior) result, when paired with the observed data. The *uniform distribution* with domain (0,1) is a special case of the beta distribution with a = b = 1. In this case, with the prior sample size a+b = 2, the data (x, n) will be the dominating factor for the posterior, and the prior is called a *flat, vague, or noninformative prior* in the Bayesian framework. We review more properties of the beta distribution and how to elicit the (a, b) hyperparameters from the investigator in Section 7.1.4.

For a given set of shape parameters (a, b), the probability $\Pr(\theta > \theta^* | x$ out of n) in Equation 7.2 can be obtained by using the R function pbeta(q, shape1, shape2). To find the usage and a numerical example, simply type the following in R:

```
> help(pbeta)
```

Example 7.1

Continuing to use the stem cell transplantation trial in Section 7.1.2 as an example, let $\theta^* = 0.15$ be the predefined threshold value. We would like to evaluate the risk of early mortality for the therapy at an interim stage when data (x, n) is available by calculating the (posterior) probability $p = \Pr(\theta > 0.15 | (x, n))$ and comparing it against a threshold, say, 80%. Suppose that we have no prior information regarding the death rate of the tested stem cell transplantation therapy. This translates to the noninformative prior, that is, beta(1,1). After experimenting on n = 5 patients, x = 1 early death occurred. The posterior $(\theta | x, n)$ ~ beta(a+x, b+n−x) = beta(2, 5). Calculate $p = \Pr(\theta > 0.15 | x = 1, n = 5)$ in R:

```
> 1-pbeta(0.15, 2, 5)
[1] 0.7764843
```

Because this answer is lower than 80%, we do not stop the study at this interim stage. (However, we would stop the study if the threshold were 0.75. For safety analysis, there is no general rule for choosing a threshold.) Note that, for a nonstatistician, 1 death out of 5 patients seems greater than a rate of 0.15. However, the calculation of probability takes into account random variation and clinicians' prior beliefs. When the trial continues, the current posterior beta(2, 5) will then become the

prior with a = 2, b = 5 for the next evaluation when a different cohort of
(x, n) is available. We can also use the same noninformative prior and
accumulate the new data (x, n) instead of a = 2, b = 5.

Figure 7.1 illustrates the noninformative prior beta(1,1) = U(0,1) modified
by the point mass data (concentrated at the point 1/5) leading to the posterior beta(2, 5).

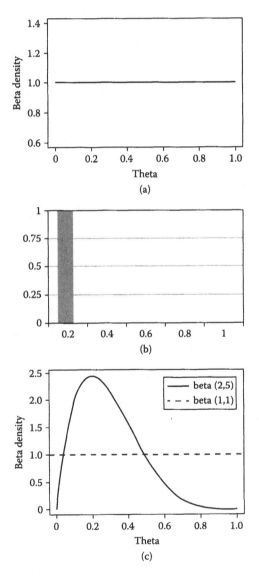

FIGURE 7.1
Posterior (c) is prior (a) modified by the data (b).

7.1.4 Elicitation of the Shape Parameters (a, b) of Beta Distribution

When the investigator has prior information on the event rate from the beginning of the trial, the noninformative prior is no longer suitable. Some soliciting methods to obtain the appropriate hyperparameters (a, b) are given by Wu, Shih, and Moore (2008). It is useful to plot the pdf f(θ; a, b) of beta(a, b), $0 \leq θ \leq 1, a > 0, b > 0$, for several possible values of (a, b) and use them during the solicitation discussion with the investigator. As an illustration, the pdf f(θ; a, b) of beta(a, b) for a = 5, b = 11 can easily be graphed in R by entering

```
t <- seq(0,1,by = 0.01)
pdf <- dbeta(t,5,11)
plot(t,pdf,type = "l",xlab = "Theta",ylab = "Beta
  density",lwd = 2)
```

Note that the mean of beta(a, b) is a/(a+b) and the mode m = (a–1)/(a+b–2). For 1 < a < b, the pdf skews to the left, such that the mode is less than the mean and both are less than 0.5 (see the example plot in Figure 7.2).

Wu, Shih, and Moore (2008) recommended two soliciting methods to obtain the appropriate hyperparameters (a, b): Method A is a "location and interval" method, and Method B is a "percentiles only" method. For both methods, we draw some rough beta distributions (pdf) during the discussion with the investigator about his/her prior beliefs (or available prior data) by performing the following:

- Method A: Elicit from the investigator the mode m (the location); select the highest density interval (r_1, r_2) and ask the investigator for the coverage probability u (area) under the pdf curve between (r_1, r_2).

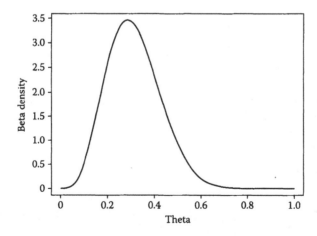

FIGURE 7.2
Density function of a beta distribution.

Given the above information, we are able to determine the parameters (a, b) of the beta prior by solving the following two equations,

$$\frac{a-1}{a+b-2} = m$$

and

$$\int_{r_1}^{r_2} f(r;a,b)dr = u \tag{7.5}$$

where $f(r;a,b) = \dfrac{\Gamma(a+b)}{\Gamma(a)\Gamma(b)} r^{a-1}(1-r)^{b-1}$ is the pdf of beta(a, b). For Method A (mode and interval), a > 1, b > 1 and $r_1 < m < r_2$. An R function, MI(m, r1, r2, u), is provided in Appendix 7.1 for obtaining the parameters (a, b).

- Method B: Give a lower percentile K_1 (100 μ_1%) and an upper percentile K_2 (100 μ_2%), and elicit from the investigator the values μ_1 and μ_2, respectively. With the information of two percentiles, K_1 and K_2, accompanying the corresponding probabilities, μ_1 and μ_2, the beta parameters can then be obtained from the numerical solution of

$$\int_0^{K_1} f(r;a,b)dr = \mu_1$$

and

$$\int_0^{K_2} f(r;a,b)dr = \mu_2 \tag{7.6}$$

For Method B (percentiles only), a ≥ 1. An R program, PO(K1, u1, K2, u2), is provided in Appendix 7.2 for obtaining the parameters (a, b).

Wu, Shih, and Moore (2008) found that when the misspecification error in judging the mode is mild, Method A is favored over Method B. The reverse is true when the error is severe.

7.1.5 Discussion

Using the posterior probability is a Bayesian approach, which enables us to incorporate expert opinion (or prior data) when making inferences and decisions. Of course, this capability is not limited to monitoring SAEs. The method can also be used for monitoring other types of events, including efficacy events (see Homework 7.1).

Some trials incorporate prior information, but utilize it in a different way. For example, one multiple myeloma trial (Montefiore-Einstein Cancer Center 2011) has the following monitoring design described in its protocol (p. 49): "The anticipated treatment related mortality with the proposed regimen is less than 5% based on previous studies.... We will consider a 30-day mortality of more than 5% as unacceptable. The 30-day mortality will be evaluated after the first 20 patients have been enrolled. If no more than 1 patient suffers a mortality within 30 days ... we will continue to accrue.... If 2 or more patients suffer a mortality ... within 30 days of treatment, we will suspend accrual...." Apparently, this study set a stopping rule of 1/20 = 0.05 as compared to the threshold based on the literature for monitoring the study, instead of using the literature to construct a prior distribution. The monitoring design thus failed to consider any variability associated with the observed data. Furthermore, with the concern of an SAE, such as 30-day mortality, a continuous monitoring plan, for example every 5 patients, seems to be more desirable than waiting for a decision when n = 20. As a homework assignment, we ask readers to use the Bayesian approach to develop a continuous safety monitoring plan (Homework 7.2).

7.1.6 Monitoring Rare Serious Events by Gamma-Poisson Distribution

The monitoring of treatment-related 30-day mortality in the multiple myeloma trial discussed above (Montefiore-Einstein Cancer Center 2011) might also be considered in another framework as a rare but serious event, if the event rate is measured in terms of per patient-month (or other continuous timescale). When using events per patient-time for a rare event, the sampling distribution for the number of events would follow a Poisson distribution with a mean rate parameter (say, λ), rather than a binomial distribution. The likelihood function is

$$\prod_{i=1}^{n} \frac{e^{-(t_i)}(t_i)^{x_i}}{x_i!}, \text{ which is proportional to } \lambda^k e^{-\lambda T} \quad \lambda > 0, T > 0, k = 0,1,2, \ldots$$

where $k = \sum_{i=1}^{n} x_i$ is the total number of events and $T = \sum_{i=1}^{n} t_i$ is the total patient-time of the sample of n subjects. The conjugate prior for λ in the Bayesian analysis would be a gamma distribution, gamma(a, b). The gamma distribution is a two-parameter family of continuous probability distributions with a shape parameter a and a rate parameter b (both > 0):

$$\text{gamma(a, b) has pdf: } f(\lambda; a, b) = \frac{b^a}{\Gamma(a)} \lambda^{a-1} e^{-\lambda b} \quad \lambda > 0$$

where $\Gamma(a)$ is the *gamma function*. A gamma density can easily be graphed by the R function *dgamma*, for example (Figure 7.3):

```
> t <- seq(0,1,by = 0.01)
> pdf <- dgamma(t,shape = 5,rate = 100)
> plot(t,pdf,type = "l",xlab = "Lambda",ylab = "Gamma
density",lwd = 2)
```

To find the prior parameters, we can elicit the prior by using the values of the mean and variance:

$$E(\lambda) = a/b$$

$$Var(\lambda) = a/b^2$$

or by methods similar to Method A ("location and interval" method) or Method B ("percentiles only" method), which were discussed for the beta distribution case. The parameter, a, represents the number of events and b represents the total patient-time.

The posterior distribution is thus, the gamma(k+a, T+b) distribution, whose pdf is proportional to

$$\lambda^{k+a-1}e^{-\lambda(T+b)}$$

We can then set a cutoff rate, λ^*, to stop the trial for safety when the posterior probability meets a threshold level of the SAE rate, for example at, 80%:

$$Pr(\lambda \geq \lambda^* \mid k, T, a, b) \geq 80\%$$

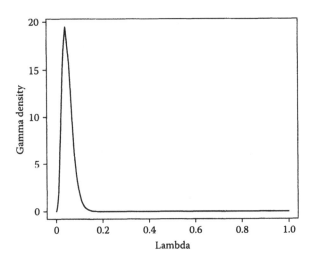

FIGURE 7.3
Density function of a gamma distribution.

Example 7.2

A completed suicide event rate in a population suffering from major depression is estimated at about 2%. In conducting a trial with a similar population, the investigator would like to stop the study if the investigational treatment group demonstrates a (true) completed suicide rate greater than 2%. The prior was determined using data from a previous study, which had four events out of 200 patient-months. In the current ongoing trial, there are two events out of 50 patient-months: should the study be stopped?

By using the Poisson-Gamma model, the estimates of prior parameters are $a = 4$ and $b = 200$; the current data is $k = 2$ and $T = 50$. The posterior is gamma(λ; 6, 250). We calculate the posterior probability $Pr(\lambda > 0.02 \mid k+a = 6, T+b = 250)$ by the R function:

```
> 1-pgamma(0.02,shape = 6,rate = 250)
[1] 0.6159607
```

Depending on the prespecified threshold level, the study may be stopped (for a threshold of, say, 60%) or not stopped (for threshold of, say, 80%).

7.2 Monitoring Futility with Conditional Probability

The Bayesian posterior probability is a conditional probability given the data. With the assistance of a prior distribution we used the Bayesian approach to monitor the safety without using significance tests. In this section, we discuss the use of conditional probability to monitor the possible *futility* of a study without a prior distribution or a p-value.

In Chapter 6, we discussed two-stage Simon's designs, where a Phase II cancer trial may be stopped at the first stage if the result is not as good as expected (desired). In that scenario, we accepted the null hypothesis and dismissed the compound from further testing to save resources and prevent more patients from being treated by an ineffective therapy. This is also known as "stopping the trial for futility." In Simon's design, the consideration was to use a least sample size while preserving the type I and type II error rates. The following conditional probability approach, on the other hand, is a monitoring tool, which does not necessarily control the type I and type II error rates.

7.2.1 Two-Stage Monitoring Process

Monitoring futility can be performed by the conditional probability (CP) method in a (classical) non-Bayesian fashion. The idea is illustrated as follows: Suppose that our final analysis is a z-test based on a total of N observations ($n = N/2$ in each treatment group for equal allocation), denoted as Z_N.

Suppose at the end of the trial we compare it to the critical value 1.96, which is the critical value for the significance level of 0.025 for a one-sided z-test. At the interim stage, we have a total of $N_1 = 2n_1$ observations, and can obtain Z_{N1}. We then (naturally) ask, what will be the probability of having the final test $Z_N > 1.96$? That is, we would like to evaluate the conditional probability, $P(Z_N > 1.96 \mid Z_{N1})$. If this probability is low, then we might stop the trial for futility.

For example, suppose we plan a trial with a total sample size of $N = 100$. When we have data for 50 patients, we calculate the z-test based on the results of these 50 patients and get $Z_{50} = 1.0$. What is $\Pr(Z_{100} > 1.96 \mid Z_{50} = 1.0)$? It turns out that the answer depends on certain factors, as follows:

Let the information time (fraction) be $t = N_1/N$. For the two-sample case, following the setting in Chapter 4 (Section 4.2), $H_0: \Delta = \mu_1 - \mu_2 = 0$, and assuming known equal within-group variance, it is straightforward to derive that

$$Z_N = \sqrt{t}Z_{N_1} + \sqrt{1-t}Z_{N-N_1} \qquad (7.7)$$

(see Appendix 7.3.1). That is, we decompose the final test statistic into two parts, one test statistic based on the samples of the first stage and one based on the rest. Note that Z_N is a weighted average of two independent normal random variables. (A linear combination of normal random variables is still normal.) The weights correspond to the square root of the sample size fraction, t, contained in each Z statistic. Specifically,

$$Z_{N_1} = \sqrt{\frac{N_1}{4\sigma^2}}\hat{\Delta} = \frac{\sqrt{N_1}\hat{\Delta}}{2\sigma} \sim N\left(\frac{\sqrt{N_1}\Delta}{2\sigma}, 1\right) \qquad (7.8)$$

$$Z_{N-N_1} \sim N\left(\frac{\sqrt{N-N_1}\Delta}{2\sigma}, 1\right)$$

and

$$Z_N \sim N\left(\frac{\sqrt{N}\Delta}{2\sigma}, 1\right) \qquad (7.9)$$

$$P\left(Z_N > 1.96 \mid Z_{N_1}\right)$$

$$= P\left(\sqrt{t}Z_{N_1} + \sqrt{1-t}Z_{N-N_1} > 1.96\right)$$

$$= P\left(Z_{N-N_1} > \frac{1.96 - \sqrt{t}Z_{N_1}}{\sqrt{1-t}}\right)$$

$$= P\left(Z_{N-N_1} - \frac{\sqrt{N-N_1}\Delta}{2\sigma} > \frac{1.96 - \sqrt{t}Z_{N_1}}{\sqrt{1-t}} - \frac{\sqrt{N-N_1}\Delta}{2\sigma} \right)$$

We use the decomposition (Equation 7.7) to calculate the CP:

$$= 1 - \Phi\left(\frac{1.96 - \sqrt{t}Z_{N_1}}{\sqrt{1-t}} - \frac{\sqrt{N-N_1}\Delta}{2\sigma} \right) \tag{7.10}$$

From Equation 7.10 we can see that the CP of the one-sided final test being significant at the 0.025 level depends not only on the interim result Z_{N_1}, but also on when the interim analysis is performed in terms of t and the true treatment effect, Δ/σ. There are many possibilities for the Δ. A pessimistic estimate of the CP is to adopt the null hypothesis, $\Delta = 0$. An optimistic estimate is to adopt the alternative hypothesis, Δ, for which the study is powered. Somewhere in between the null and alternative hypothesis is the point estimate of Δ based on the interim data and the assumption that the current trend will continue to the end of the trial. Another estimate may be the upper or lower limit of a confidence interval. Moreover, one can make a weighted average of the above choices. If we place a (prior) distribution for Δ, with a certain degree of variability centered at the point estimate and, for example, averaging Equation 7.10 with respect to this (prior) distribution, we then obtain a predictive probability of the one-sided final test being significant.

The point estimate of Δ with the interim data is seen in Equation 7.8:

$$\hat{\Delta} = \frac{2\sigma}{\sqrt{N_1}} Z_{N_1} \tag{7.11}$$

Thus, set $\Delta = \hat{\Delta}$ in (7.10) and, since $\frac{N-N_1}{N_1} = \frac{1-t}{t}$, we obtain

$$CP\left(Z_{N_1}, t, \text{current trend} \right) = 1 - \Phi\left(\frac{1.96 - \sqrt{t}Z_{N_1}}{\sqrt{1-t}} - \sqrt{\frac{1-t}{t}}Z_{N_1} \right)$$

$$= \Phi\left(\frac{Z_{N_1}}{\sqrt{t(1-t)}} - \frac{1.96}{\sqrt{1-t}} \right) \tag{7.12}$$

Equation 7.12 can also be derived from the familiar regression formula of a bivariate normal distribution; see Appendix 7.3.3. Continuing the example where we supposed $Z_{N_1} = 1.0$ at $t = 50/100 = 1/2$, under the current trend, $CP = \Phi\left(2 - 1.96\sqrt{2} \right) = 0.22$ by the R function:

```
> pnorm(2-1.96*sqrt(2))
[1] 0.2200991
```

If the threshold for the CP is set at 0.30 in the monitoring plan, then the study would be stopped for futility.

In-Class Exercises

1. What would be the CP if the same Z-value ($Z_{N_1} = 1.0$) was observed at an earlier or later information time fraction, say t = 1/3 or 2/3?
2. What Z-value would one need to have at an interim analysis for the CP to be at least 50%, assuming that the current trend will continue? The answer should be a function of t.

7.2.2 Discussion

Some points with regard to early termination require further attention. First, stopping the study for futility means that the compound (or concept) is dismissed from further testing in this study. This action does not necessarily mean that the sponsoring company or the investigator would abandon the compound completely. The compound may be modified for the dose regimen, route of administration, combined with other compounds, or studied for other indications with other populations.

Second, performing an interim analysis affects the type I error rate. As we previously demonstrated with Simon's two-stage design, when the interim analysis stops the trial only for futility, the type I error rate will be deflated, as also shown algebraically:

$$\alpha = P_0(\text{Reject } H_0)$$

$$= P_0(\text{Not stop at } t < 1 \text{ then, reject } H_0 \text{ at } t = 1)$$

$$< P_0(\text{reject } H_0 \text{ at } t = 1)$$

$$= P_0(Z_N > 1.96) = 0.025$$

Normally, this suggests that one can set the critical value less than 1.96 for the final analysis to be significant at the 5% level for a two-sided test or the 2.5% level for a one-sided test, which is quite a gain. However, this is not a practice permitted by the FDA for Phase III pivotal studies in the NDA setting, because the regulatory agency (rightly) regards the futility rule as not enforceable, that is, nonbinding to the company. Provided that it is not a safety issue, the company may not adhere to the futility rule and still continue the study despite the low CP, which, although unwise, is nevertheless a business decision.

Appendix 7.1: R Function for Obtaining Parameters of Prior Distribution Beta(a, b) Based on Method A

Gives the mode (m) and the coverage probability (u) of an interval (r1, r2).

The R Function MI (Mode and Interval Method)

```
# programmed by Yujun Wu; see Wu, Shih and Moore (2008)
# r1 < m < r2
###########################################################
# Method A: Location (mode) and Interval
# Elicitation information: (1) mode m
#                          (2) Pr(r1<r<r2) = u
###########################################################

MI <- function(m, r1, r2, u) {

  S <- function(x){
    (pbeta(r2,x[1],x[2])-pbeta(r1,x[1],x[2])-u)^2 +((x[1]-1)/
      (x[1]+x[2]-2)-m)^2
  }
  obj = constrOptim(c(2,2), S, NULL, ui = rbind(c(1,0),c(0,1)),
    ci = c(1,1), mu = 1e-100, outer.eps = 1e-100)
  obj$par
}
# Example:
MI(0.05,0.01,0.10,0.8)
```

Appendix 7.2: R Function for Obtaining Parameters of Prior Distribution Beta(a, b) Based on Method B

Gives the lower (100u1%) percentile (K1) and the (100u2%) percentile (K2).

The R Function MI (Percentiles Only Method)

```
# programmed by Yujun Wu; see Wu, Shih and Moore (2008)
# K1 < K2
###########################################################
# Method B: percentiles only
# Elicitation information: (1) K1 : Pr(r<K1) = u1
#                          (2) K2 : Pr(r<K2) = u2
###########################################################
```

```
PO <- function(K1,u1,K2,u2) {

  S <- function(x) {
    (pbeta(K1,x[1],x[2])-u1)^2 +(pbeta(K2,x[1],x[2])-u2)^2
  }
  obj = constrOptim(c(2,2), S, NULL, ui = rbind(c(1,0),c(0,1)),
    ci = c(1,1), mu = 1e-100, outer.eps = 1e-100)
  obj$par
}

# Example:
PO(0.05, 0.90, 0.15, 0.99)
```

Appendix 7.3: Notes on the Two-Stage Monitoring Process

Appendix 7.3.1

Any process S_m that is a sum of m identically independently distributed (iid) random variables W_i (i = 1 to m), $S_m = \sum_1^m W_i$, can also be written as a sum of two independent partial sums, $S_m = S_{m1} + S_{m-m1}$ for $m_1 < m$. Furthermore, with the assumption of finite variances for W_i, by the central limit theorem, $\sqrt{m}(S_m/m)$ is asymptotically normally distributed and so are the component partial sums with sample sizes m_1 and $m-m_1$, respectively. Hence, without loss of generality, we consider the z-test statistics for comparing two treatment groups with equal sample size and common within-group variance σ^2 and equal accrual rate, and express the following for any independent partial sum process. Let n = N/2 and $n_1 = N_1/2$.

Specifically, for testing difference in means, let $\bar{X}_n \sim N(\mu_x, \sigma^2/n)$, $\bar{Y}_n \sim N(\mu_y, \sigma^2/n)$, $Z_N = \frac{1}{\sqrt{2\sigma}} \sqrt{n}(\bar{X}_n - \bar{Y}_n)$ and $Z_{N_1} = \frac{1}{\sqrt{2\sigma}} \sqrt{n_1}(\bar{X}_{n_1} - \bar{Y}_{n_1})$. Then

$$Z_N = \frac{1}{\sqrt{2\sigma}} \frac{1}{\sqrt{n}} \left(\sum_{i=1}^n X_i - \sum_{i=1}^n Y_i \right)$$

$$= \frac{1}{\sqrt{2\sigma}} \left[\frac{1}{\sqrt{n}} \right] \left[\sqrt{n_1} \left(\frac{\sum_1^{n_1} X_i - \sum_1^{n_1} Y_i}{\sqrt{n_1}} \right) + \sqrt{n-n_1} \left(\frac{\sum_{n_1+1}^n X_i - \sum_{n_1+1}^n Y_i}{\sqrt{n-n_1}} \right) \right]$$

$$= \sqrt{N_1/N}\, Z_{N_1} + \sqrt{(N-N_1)/N}$$

$$= \sqrt{t} Z_{N_1} + \sqrt{1-t} Z_{N-N_1}$$

with t = $N_1/N = n_1/n$. (This is Equation 7.7.)

Notice that $Z_N = \sqrt{n/2}\,\Delta/\sigma$, $E(Z_{N_1}) = \sqrt{n_1/2}\,\Delta/\sigma$, $\mathrm{Var}(Z_N) = \mathrm{Var}(Z_{N_1}) = 1$ and $\mathrm{Cov}(Z_N, Z_{N_1}) = \mathrm{Cov}(\sqrt{t}Z_{N_1} + \sqrt{1-t}Z_{N-N_1}, Z_{N_1}) = \sqrt{t}$. These characterize the joint distribution of (Z_N, Z_{N_1}).

Appendix 7.3.2

The above equation $Z_N = \sqrt{t}Z_{N_1} + \sqrt{1-t}Z_{N-N}$, for $t = N_1/N = n_1/n$, can be generalized to $Z_W = w_1 Z_{N_1} + w_2 Z_{N-N_1}$ for any weights $(w_1, w_2) > (0, 0)$ with $w_1^2 + w_2^2 = 1$. We can also express the Z-value by its corresponding p-value: $Z_w = \Phi^{-1}(1-p) = w_1\Phi^{-1}(1 - p_1) + w_2\Phi^{-1}(1 - p_2)$. Hence a further extension of the final test is to combine the p-values (p_1, p_2) of the two stages: $1 - p = \Phi[w_1\Phi^{-1}(1 - p_1) + w_2\Phi^{-1}(1 - p_2)]$. The advantage of this extension is that the p-values of the two stages can be obtained by different tests or different endpoints when necessary. For example, the first endpoint for an interim analysis could be a surrogate endpoint, and the final test could be based on a clinical endpoint. When there is a multiple comparison situation, the p-values at the two stages could also be the adjusted p-values. For example, if the first stage involves dose selection among several candidate doses, and the second stage compares the winning dose with the control agent, then the first stage can have an adjusted p-value from one of the step-down or step-up methods. The generalization to more than two stages is also apparent. However, if the weights are too arbitrary or weighs too differently for observations at different stages, the weighted test Z_W can lose efficiency or even become peculiar.

Appendix 7.3.3

In this section we review of the basic formulas for the bivariate normal distribution, simple linear regression, and application to the derivation of the CP (Equation 7.10). Let (X,Y) have a bivariate normal distribution, with $E(Y) = \mu_Y$, $E(X) = \mu_X$, $\mathrm{Var}(Y) = \sigma_Y^2$, $\mathrm{Var}(X) = \sigma_X^2$, and $\mathrm{Corr}(Y,X) = \rho$, $0 < |\rho| < 1$. The simple linear regression has $E(Y\mid X) = \mu_Y - \rho\dfrac{\sigma_Y}{\sigma_X}(X - \mu_X)$, and $\mathrm{Var}(Y\mid X) = \sigma_Y^2(1 - \rho^2)$. Therefore,

$$E(Z_N \mid Z_{N_1}) = E(Z_N) - \sqrt{t}\left(Z_{N_1} - E(Z_{N_1})\right)$$

$$= \sqrt{n/2}\,\Delta/\sigma - \sqrt{t}\left(Z_{N_1} - \sqrt{n_1/2}\,\Delta/\sigma\right)$$

and
$$\mathrm{Var}(Z_N \mid Z_{N_1}) = 1 - t$$

When we substitute the estimate $\hat{\Delta} = \dfrac{2\sigma}{\sqrt{N_1}}Z_{N_1} = \dfrac{\sqrt{2}\sigma}{\sqrt{n_1}}Z_{N_1}$ as in Equation 7.11, we have

$$E(Z_N \mid Z_{N_1}) = \sqrt{n/n_1}Z_{N_1} - \sqrt{t}\left(Z_{N_1} - Z_{N_1}\right) = \sqrt{1/t}Z_{N_1}$$

Therefore, $P\left(Z_N > 1.96 \mid Z_{N_1}, \text{current trend}\right)$

$$= 1 - \Phi\left(\frac{1.96 - \sqrt{1/t}\,Z_{N_1}}{\sqrt{1-t}}\right)$$

$$= \Phi\left(\frac{Z_{N_1}}{\sqrt{t(1-t)}} - \frac{1.96}{\sqrt{1-t}}\right)$$

Homework 7.1

A pilot study was conducted to evaluate the impact of green tea extract in patients with indolent chronic lymphocytic leukemia (CLL) or low-grade non-Hodgkin's lymphoma (NHL) who are not receiving cytotoxic therapy (Strair et al. 2005). The primary endpoints were toxicity and disease impact. The protocol described the following monitoring plan: Patients are monitored every 4 months while taking green tea extract, and each clinical evaluation will be scored as stable disease, clinically improved (complete response + partial response), or progressive disease. The study will accrue up to 24 patients. It will be discontinued if the investigating team is at least 80% certain that fewer than 15% of patients have a clinically improved response (futility) or if the team is at least 90% certain that more than 30% of patients will progress within 1 year (toxicity and futility). You are asked to formulate a statistical strategy to set up the stopping rule when patients are sequentially observed over the study period.

> Make two tables of posterior probabilities that display the stopping rule. The tables can be made with spreadsheets: the rows are numbers of patients (sample size at the time of monitoring) and the columns are numbers of patients with event. Inside the tables display the posterior probabilities. Use a noninformative prior distribution. (Writing an SAS or R program will make your job much easier.)

> After constructing the tables, make clear instructions and highlight the tables (e.g., with shade or color) to direct the team regarding the stopping rule.

> Note that these two tables should only be used for the first monitoring stage. The following monitoring stages should use updated beta priors based on the observations in the previous stages.

Homework 7.2

For the multiple myeloma trial (Montefiore-Einstein Cancer Center 2011), use the Bayesian approach to develop a continuous safety monitoring plan. For determining the beta prior distribution on the treatment-related 30-day mortality rate, let the mode be 0.05, and the probability of mortality rate falling between 0.01 and 0.15 be 80%. Use the R program in Appendix 7.1 to find the beta parameters. Construct a table of posterior probabilities that displays the stopping rules up to n = 40. Repeat the same exercise if we narrow the interval of mortality rate to 0.01 and 0.10 for coverage probability of 80%.

References

Eastern Cooperative Oncology Group. (2001). Chemotherapy and Peripheral Stem Cell Transplantation in Treating Patients with Multiple Myeloma. ClinicalTrials. gov Identifier: NCT00014508.

EMA (European Medicines Agency). (1995). ICH Topic E 2 A: Clinical Safety Data Management: Definitions and Standards for Expedited Reporting. http://www. ema.europa.eu/docs/en_GB/document_library/Scientific_guideline/2009/09/ WC500002749.pdf

FDA (US Department of Health and Human Services Food and Drug Administration). (2007). *Guidance for Industry, Drug-Induced Liver Injury: Premarketing Clinical Evaluation Oct 2007.*

Montefiore-Einstein Cancer Center. (2011). A Phase II Study Assessing the Efficacy and Toxicity of PK-Directed Intravenous Busulfan in Combination with High-Dose Melphalan and Bortezomib as Conditioning Regimen for First-Line Autologous Hematopoietic Stem Cell Transplantation in Patients with Multiple Myeloma, Albert Einstein Cancer Center, NY. https://clinicaltrials. gov/identifier:NCT01605032

NCI (National Cancer Institute). (2009). Common Terminology Criteria for Adverse Events. http://evs.nci.nih.gov/ftp1/CTCAE/CTCAE_4.03_2010-06-14_Quick Reference_5x7.pdf (accessed March 18, 2014).

Strair R, Rubin A, Bertino J, Schaar D, Gharibo M, Goodin S, Krimmel T, et al. (2005). Green Tea for Patients with Indolent Non-Hodgkin's Lymphoma or Chronic Lymphocytic Leukemia not Receiving Cytotoxic Therapy. The Cancer Institute of New Jersey, New Brunswick, NJ.

Wu Y, Shih WJ, and Moore DF. (2008). Elicitation of a beta prior for Bayesian inference in clinical trials. *Biometrical Journal* 50: 212–223.

8

Sequential Designs and Methods—Part III: Classical Group Sequential Trials

In Chapters 6 and 7, we discussed two-stage designs. Group sequential design is a generalization for multiple stage designs. The classical group sequential procedure (design, monitoring, and analysis) is probably the most commonly applied method to facilitate the conduct of interim analysis in clinical trials, especially trials with mortality or severe or irreversible morbidity as the primary endpoints. In clinical trials with such endpoints, the fundamental consideration is an ethical obligation to modify or terminate the study at the earliest opportunity to prevent administration of a less favorable (for efficacy or toxicity) therapy to additional patients. Conducting these clinical trials in stages, with group evaluation sizes predetermined by a certain schedule, provides logistical feasibility over fully sequential methods, because the endpoint in these trials can often take a long time to occur. However, the advantage of reducing the average sample number still applies. Many different methods for group sequential procedures are available and include different stopping boundaries, different type I error spending/use functions, conditional or predictive power approaches, Bayesian methods, etc. These procedures are based on a *fixed maximum sample size*. We call them *classical group sequential methods* to distinguish them from the more recent development in using *adaptive group sequential methods*, in which one can extend the maximum sample size or modify other design specifications, such as study population or endpoint, as the trial is ongoing. With more flexibility and potential of introducing bias by monitoring interim data, regulatory authorities have developed strict guidance, particularly for group sequential trials. The logistics of a group sequential trial are also complicated and require careful planning and execution.

8.1 Regulatory Requirements and Logistical Considerations for Trial Monitoring

The International Conference on Harmonisation *Guidelines for Industry* (ICH 1998) discuss regulatory requirements on interim analyses in general (E3, Section 11.4.2.3) and group sequential procedures in particular, regarding data monitoring and early stopping (E9, Sections 3.4 and 4.1–4.6). The following is a summary (Shih 2000):

- All interim analyses should be carefully planned in advance and fully described in the protocol. Unplanned interim analyses should be avoided if at all possible. In the event that an unplanned interim analysis was conducted, a protocol amendment describing the interim analysis should be completed prior to unblinded access to treatment comparison data. In addition, the study report should also explain the necessity of the interim analysis, the degree to which the blindness will be broken, and provide an assessment of the potential magnitude of bias introduced as well as the impact on the interpretation of the results.

- The schedule of analyses, or at least the considerations that will govern the generation of the interim analysis, should be stated in the protocol or amendment before the time of the first interim analysis; the stopping guidelines and their properties should also be clearly stated there.

- The procedure plan should be written or approved by the data monitoring committee (DMC), when the trial has one.

- Any changes to the trial and any consequent changes to the statistical procedures should be specified in an amendment to the protocol at the earliest opportunity.

- The procedures selected should always ensure that the overall probability of the type I error is controlled.

- The execution of an interim analysis must be a completely confidential process when unblinded data and results are potentially involved. All staff involved in the conduct of the trial should remain blinded to the results of such analyses. Investigators should only be informed about the decision to continue or discontinue the trial, or to implement modifications to trial procedures.

- Any interim analysis planned for administrative purposes only should also be described in the protocol and subsequently reported. Examples include speeding up recruitment, updating trial progress for stakeholders, etc. The specific purposes should be clearly stated and should specifically exclude any possibility of early stopping. In these circumstances, the blinding should not be broken.

The organization of a trial conduct and data monitoring is an important part of the study design. Figure 8.1 illustrates the four components of a trial organization, involving the trial sponsor (e.g., industry, NIH); investigators;

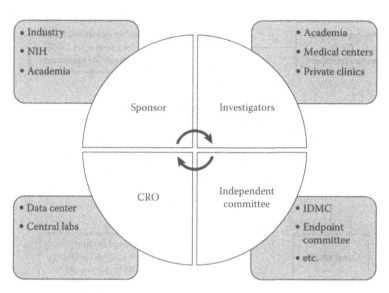

FIGURE 8.1
Four components of a trial organization.

contract research organization (CRO), which manages the database and issues reports to the DMC according to an agreed schedule; and independent committees, including a DMC and, if necessary, an endpoint adjudication committee (EAC), etc. The separation of these components is specifically designed to install checks and balances to prevent potential operational bias.

Read the article in Homework 8.1 for an example of a trial with detailed organization and study schedules in the design section.

The primary obligation of the DMC is to protect the safety of the patients in the trial. In many trials, the DMC is also charged with monitoring the efficacy of the study medications according to the DMC charter. Safety must ultimately be monitored with respect to the risk–benefit ratio; thus efficacy cannot be ignored in the whole picture of the DMC's function. In addition, the DMC often also focuses on ongoing accrual and the trial and data integrity as a service to those subjects who enrolled in anticipation of completing and answering the study question. Usually, the DMC is organized with members from institutions external to the sponsor and investigators; it is supposed to make independent recommendations to the sponsor through an executive committee or sponsor committee, thus it is also known as an independent DMC or IDMC. The DMC also includes an independent statistician and often a patient advocate. A functional flowchart of the DMC is illustrated in Figure 8.2. A good discussion on IDMC is given by Ellenberg (2001).

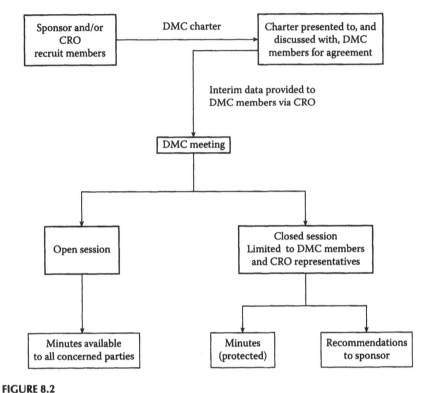

FIGURE 8.2
IDMC's process.

8.2 Statistical Methods

8.2.1 Fundamentals

Let us start by considering the design of a clinical trial with a plan of monitoring the data at calendar times ct_1, ct_2, ..., ct_K for some fixed $K > 1$. For example, a trial monitoring committee might plan to meet every April 1 and October 1 for the first 2 years and then every June 15 for the rest of the trial duration. The amount of information at the calendar time provided by the data can be considered as an idea of *generalized sample size*. Mathematically, it refers to the (observed) *Fisher information* and it is used for obtaining the statistic in the *score test*. (See Appendices 4.1 through 4.4 of Chapter 4). In estimation, the variance of an estimator is the inverse of the Fisher information, and vice versa. For continuous and binary endpoints, information is proportional to the subject count (what we called sample size before.)

This is seen by using $\bar{X}_n - \bar{Y}_n$ to estimate the treatment mean difference Δ. With $\mathrm{Var}(\bar{X}_n - \bar{Y}_n) = \dfrac{2\sigma^2}{n}$, the information equals $\dfrac{n}{2\sigma^2}$. Appendices 4.1

through 4.4 of Chapter 4 also showed that, for time-to-event (survival) endpoints, information is proportional to the event count. By a similar derivation with likelihood functions, we can show that, for a longitudinal analysis, information is proportional to the number of visits (e.g., subject-months for calculating the exposure experience), which is a special case of correlated (clustered) data in general. From Chapter 4, Section 4.5, we can see that for clustered data, information is proportional to the sub-unit and whole-unit counts together. When we are dealing with a process with time, we then denote the information at calendar time ct_i as I_i and the fixed total/maximum information at ct_K as I_{max}. The corresponding $ti = Ii/Imax$ at ct_i, $i = 1, \ldots, K$, are the information times (or *information fractions*). Note that $t_K = 1$. When information is proportional to the sample size, then $t_i = Ii/Imax = N_i/N_{max}$. This coincides with the notation we previously used in Chapter 6, where we only considered two stages. Because the information time is just a rescaled calendar time, we sometimes write $I(t_i) = I_i$ for convenience.

At information time t_i, $i = 1, \ldots, K$, standardized Z-statistics, $Z_{t_1}, Z_{t_2}, \ldots, Z_{t_k}$ are calculated based on the accumulated data for testing hypotheses about the treatment effect represented by a parameter θ. A focal statistical problem of the group sequential procedures is to find critical values to satisfy certain desirable operational characteristics. These critical values are termed *group sequential boundaries*. For example, for a one-sided hypothesis with the decision options being "either reject H_0: $\theta = 0$ or continue at the interim stages," and "reject or accept H_0 at the final stage," the problem is to find values $b_1, b_2, \ldots, b_K$ such that the overall type I error rate α is maintained at a prespecified level α:

$$P_{H_0}(\text{Reject } H_0) = P_{H_0}(Z_{t_1} \geq b_1 \text{ or } Z_{t_2} \geq b_2 \text{ or} \ldots Z_{t_k} \geq b_K) = \alpha \qquad (8.1)$$

Finding the critical values $b_1, b_2, \ldots, b_K$ is necessary because, for example, Armitage, McPherson, and Rowe (1969) showed that for $K > 1$, if the critical values at the interim stages remain at 1.96, then

$$P_{H_0}(Z_{t_1} \geq 1.96 \text{ or } Z_{t_2} \geq 1.96 \text{ or } \ldots Z_{t_k} \geq 1.96) > 0.025$$

Table 8.1 gives more cases of inflation of type I error rate by repeated testing of H_0 with the same critical value without proper adjustment for the nominal level of error rate at $\alpha = 0.01, 0.02,$ or 0.05.

Equation 8.1 uses a one-sided test for easy illustration. For a corresponding two-sided hypothesis test, a symmetric boundary would replace α with $\alpha/2$ then apply the one-sided boundary symmetrically to the lower boundary. Asymmetric boundaries also have been proposed in the literature (e.g., DeMets and Ware 1982), however, they are seldom used in a regulatory NDA setting. In the following we consider several commonly cited group sequential boundaries.

TABLE 8.1

Inflation of Type I Error Rate Occurs by Repeated Testing of
H_0 with the Same Critical Value without Proper Adjustment

K	Nominal 0.05	Nominal 0.02	Nominal 0.01
1	0.05	0.02	0.01
2	0.0831	0.0345	0.0177
3	0.1072	0.0456	0.0237
4	0.1262	0.0545	0.0286
5	0.1417	0.0620	0.0327
10	0.1933	0.0877	0.0474
20	0.2479	0.1163	0.0640

8.2.2 Equally Spaced Group Sequential Boundaries

Suppose that the information times are equally spaced: $t_1 = 1/K$, $t_2 = 2/K$, ...,
$t_K = K/K = 1$. In the 1970s, Haybittle (1971) and Peto et al. (1976), Pocock (1977),
and O'Brien and Fleming (1979) proposed different boundaries as follows:

- Haybittle–Peto: Find $b_i = c$ for $i = 1, ..., K - 1$ and $b_K = z_{1-\alpha}$ such that

$$P_{Ho}(Z_{t_1} \geq c \text{ or } Z_{t_2} \geq c \text{ or } ... Z_{t_k} \geq z_{1-\alpha}) = \alpha \qquad (8.2)$$

For example, if we set $\alpha = 0.025$ and $K = 5$, then $c = 3.291$. The boundaries
are (3.291, 3.291, 3.291, 3.291, 1.960).

The rationale for the Haybittle–Peto boundary was to let the critical value
of the final test be $z_{1-\alpha}$, as if it were for a fixed sample size trial, to alleviate
the perception of "alpha punishment" from clinical colleagues. However,
when the final test is at the same level as the fixed-size design, the overall
type I error rate must be inflated by tests at the interim stages. Hence, the
above example cannot be exactly correct. One can only say that the last
critical value resembles the fixed sample size design. Thus, Pocock (1977)
proposed a corrected solution as follows.

- Pocock: Find $b_i = c$ for $i = 1, ..., K$ such that

$$P_{Ho}(Z_{t_1} \geq c \text{ or } Z_{t_2} \geq c \text{ or } ... Z_{t_k} \geq c) = \alpha \qquad (8.3)$$

For example, if we set $\alpha = 0.025$ and $K = 5$, then $c = 2.413$. The boundaries
are (2.413, 2.413, 2.413, 2.413, 2.413).

The rationale for the Pocock boundary was to simplify the monitoring process by having a constant (same) critical value for all the tests. However, this
convenience ignores the fact that early tests are based on less information
than later tests. We often desire to protect the trial from being stopped too

early, unless the evidence in the data is tremendously convincing. This led to the following O'Brien-Fleming (OBF) boundary.

- OBF: Find c such that

$$P_{H_0}(Z_{t_1}\sqrt{t_1} \geq c \text{ or } Z_{t_2}\sqrt{t_2} \geq c \text{ or } \ldots Z_{t_k}\sqrt{t_k} \geq c) = \alpha \qquad (8.4)$$

For $\alpha = 0.025$ and $K = 5$, $c = 2.04$. Hence, $b_i = 2.04/\sqrt{t_i} = 2.04/\sqrt{i/5}$. The boundaries are (4.562, 3.226, 2.634, 2.281, 2.040).

Note that in Equation 8.4, it is the $Z_{t_i}\sqrt{t_i}$, not the Z-statistics themselves, that we compare to the same critical value throughout the study, in order to account for the increasing cumulative information in the data set as time goes on. The quantity $Z_{t_i}\sqrt{t_i}$ is known as the *B-value* (B for *Brownian motion*) by Lan and Wittes (1988).

Figure 8.3 depicts the above boundaries for a two-sided hypothesis. For a one-sided hypothesis H_A: $\theta > 0$, there should not be a lower boundary; only the upper boundary (with alpha = 0.025) applies. We can still use Figure 8.3, but the area below the lower boundary will then be interpreted as acceptance of H_0: $\theta \leq 0$ for considering futility with a symmetric boundary. The boundary shape shows that the OBF boundary has the characteristic that the critical value starts high in the beginning then lowers toward the end of the trial. Therefore, it is the most stringent boundary for early interim

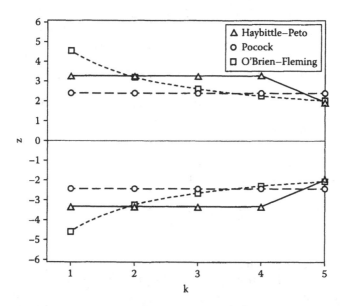

FIGURE 8.3
Three classical sequential boundaries with five analyses at equally spaced intervals, two-sided alpha = 0.05.

analyses among the three. The choice of boundary, however, should depend on the purpose or intention of using a design with early stopping rules. The calculation of the boundaries requires iterative numerical integrations.

At the design stage it may be reasonable to plan for a fixed number of K analyses at equally spaced information times. However, when the trial is ongoing and being monitored, operational changes often occur. Interim analyses might not necessarily follow the preplanned schedule, and the frequency of the analyses, K, may also change. This situation requires a more flexible procedure. Slud and Wei (1982) and Lan and DeMets (1983) developed the *type I error spending/use function* approach to meet this need.

8.2.3 Type I Error Spending/Use Function Approach

The idea of the type I error spending/use function as an approach can be illustrated as follows: We first untie the fixed K in the expression in Equation 8.1 and decompose the rejection region, R, into disjointed regions as follows:

$$R = \{Z_{t_1} \geq b_1 \text{ or } Z_{t_2} \geq b_2 \text{ or } Z_{t_3} \geq b_3 ...\}$$

Let $R_1 = \{Z_{t_1} \geq b_1\}$. Thus, $\{Z_{t_1} \geq b_1 \text{ or } Z_{t_2} \geq b_2\} = \{Z_{t_1} \geq b_1\} \cup \{Z_{t_1} < b_1, Z_{t_2} \geq b_2\} \equiv R_1 \cup R_2$, and $\{Z_{t_1} \geq b_1 \text{ or } Z_{t_2} \geq b_2 \text{ or } Z_{t_3} \geq b_3\} = (R_1 \cup R_2) \cup \{Z_{t_1} < b_1, Z_{t_2} < b_2, Z_{t_3} \geq b_3\} \equiv (R_1 \cup R_2) \cup R_3$, and so on. Hence,

$$P_{Ho}(R) = P_{Ho}(R_1 \cup R_2 \cup R_3 \cup ...)$$

$$= P_{Ho}(R_1) + P_{Ho}(R_2) + P_{Ho}(R_3) + ... = \alpha$$

At t_1 we specify a value of $\alpha(t_1) = P_{Ho}(R_1)$ and solve for b_1. At t_2, specify

$$\alpha(t_2) = P_{Ho}(R_1 \cup R_2) = P_{Ho}(R_1) + P_{Ho}(R_2) \text{ (due to disjointed regions)}$$

$$= \alpha(t_1) + P_{Ho}(R_2)$$

This leads to $P_{Ho}(R_2) = \alpha(t_2) - \alpha(t_1)$, and we can solve for b_2, since b_1 is already known from the first stage. Similarly at t_3, specify

$$\alpha(t_3) = P_{Ho}(R_1 \cup R_2 \cup R_3) = (P_{Ho}(R_1) + P_{Ho}(R_2)) + P_{Ho}(R_3)$$

$$= \alpha(t_2) + P_{Ho}(R_3)$$

Therefore, $P_{Ho}(R_3) = \alpha(t_3) - \alpha(t_2)$. We then solve for b_3, because b_1 and b_2 were already solved in the previous steps. The process continues.

Note that, when solving for b_2, we only need the joint distribution of (Z_{t_1}, Z_{t_2}). In Appendix 7.3 of Chapter 7, we introduced the idea of decomposing a sum process into two independent partial sums and derived formulas for calculating the conditional probability. Here, we generalize that idea with the generalized sample size, that is, statistical information. In a generalized term, for a *partial sum process* with *independent increments*, where we can write the score test as $Z_{t_i} = \frac{S(t_i)}{\sqrt{I(t_i)}}$, with the numerator being the cumulative sum of the observations (iid variates with mean θ) and the denominator being the square root of the cumulative statistical information in estimating θ at time t_i, the correlation is then

$$\rho(t_1, t_2) = \text{Corr} = \text{Cov}(Z_{t_1}, Z_{t_2}) = \text{Cov}\left(\frac{S(t_1)}{\sqrt{I(t_1)}}, \frac{S(t_2)}{\sqrt{I(t_2)}} \right)$$

$$= \text{Cov}\left(\frac{S(t_1)}{\sqrt{I(t_1)}}, \frac{S(t_1) + (S(t_2) - S(t_1))}{\sqrt{I(t_2)}} \right)$$

$$= \frac{1}{\sqrt{I(t_1)I(t_2)}} \text{Var}(S(t_1)) = \sqrt{\frac{I(t_1)}{I(t_2)}} = \sqrt{\frac{I(t_1)/I(t_K)}{I(t_2)/I(t_K)}} = \sqrt{\frac{t_1}{t_2}}$$

where $t_i = I(t_i)/I(t_K) = I_i/I_{max}$, as noted previously in Section 8.2.1.

Other time-point boundaries follow similarly. When information is proportional to the sample size, then $\rho(t_1, t_2) = (N_1/N_2)^{1/2} = (t_1/t_2)^{1/2}$. Therefore, the joint distribution only involves the ratio of information at the current stage and before, not the later time points. This approach allows for a great deal of flexibility when monitoring trials, because there is no requirement for K, the total number of analyses, nor is there the "equally spaced t_i" restriction. All that is needed is $\alpha(t_1) < \alpha(t_2) < \ldots < \alpha(1) = \alpha$, a strictly increasing function $\alpha(t)$, known as the *type I error (α) spending/use function*, prespecified in the study design protocol.

Example 8.1: Two-Stage Design (One Interim and One Final Analyses) With Symmetric Boundaries

Specify the overall type I error $\alpha = 0.05$ (two-sided test) and the *linear (uniform) alpha-spending function* as $\alpha(t) = \alpha t$. Suppose we conduct an interim analysis when $t_1 = 1/2$, then $\alpha(t_1 = 1/2) = 0.025$. The corresponding boundary point at $t_1 = 1/2$ is $b_1 = 2.2414$. This leaves $\alpha - \alpha(t_1 = 1/2) = 0.025$ to be spent at the final stage $t_2 = 1$. Solving $\Pr\{|Z_{t_1}| < 2.2414, |Z_{t_2}| \geq b_2\} = 0.025$ given that the correlation of the bivariate normal distribution is $\sqrt{t_1/t_2} = \sqrt{1/2}$, we obtain $b_2 = 2.1251$. (An R function to do this calculation is given in Appendix 8.1). Note that at the final stage $\alpha_2 \equiv \Pr(|Z| \geq 2.1251) = 0.0336$. That is, with this linear/uniform spending function, $\alpha(t) = \alpha t$, if an interim testing is to be conducted in the middle of the trial, the p-value at the final stage has to be less than 0.034, instead of at the 0.05 level, to be significant. This requirement often feels like a "penalty" to some clinical investigators. On the other hand, because there was $\alpha(t_1 = 1/2) = 0.025$ spent for the interim analysis, the remaining alpha available for the final analysis is $0.05 - 0.025 = 0.025$, but due to the correlation of Z_{t_1} and Z_{t_2}, the critical region for the analysis actually corresponds to alpha level of $0.0336 > 0.025$.

Following this example, a natural question arises: What kind of alpha-spending function would describe the Pocock boundary and the OBF boundary in Section 8.2.2? We look at the following example in search for an answer.

Example 8.2

$K = 5$, $\alpha = 0.025$, Pocock Boundary: (2.413, 2.413, 2.413, 2.413, 2.413)
1. With the first critical value, we can find the corresponding alpha spent at the first stage $P_{Ho}(Z_{t_1} \geq 2.413) = 0.0079$. Therefore, $\alpha(t_1 = 1/5) = 0.0079$. Next, we continue to calculate for the second stage.

2. The cumulative alpha at the second stage is $P_{Ho}(Z_{t_1} \geq 2.413$ or $Z_{t_2} \geq 2.413)$
$= P_{Ho}(Z_{t_1} \geq 2.413) + P_{Ho}(Z_{t_1} < 2.413, Z_{t_2} \geq 2.413)$
$= 0.0079 + 0.0059$
$= 0.0138$. Therefore, $\alpha(t_2 = 2/5) = 0.0138$

3. The cumulative alpha at the third stage is $P_{Ho}(Z_{t_1} \geq 2.413$ or $Z_{t_2} \geq 2.413$ or $Z_{t_3} \geq 2.413)$
$= P_{Ho}(Z_{t_1} \geq 2.413$ or $Z_{t_2} \geq 2.413) + P_{Ho}((Z_{t_1} < 2.413, Z_{t_2} < 2.413), Z_{t_3} \geq 2.413)$
$= 0.0138 + 0.0045$
$= 0.0183$. Therefore, $\alpha(t_3 = 3/5) = 0.0183$. Note that we add 0.0045, the incremental alpha, to the second stage alpha 0.0138.

4. Following similar steps, we obtain for the fourth stage cumulative alpha: $P_{Ho}(Z_{t_1} \geq 2.413$ or $Z_{t_2} \geq 2.413$ or $Z_{t_3} \geq 2.413$ or $Z_{t_4} \geq 2.413)$
$= \ldots$ (similar steps)
$= 0.0183 + 0.0036$
$= 0.0219$. Hence, $\alpha(t_4 = 4/5) = 0.0219$

5. The final stage alpha would be the total alpha $(= 0.025$ in this case), as shown:
$P_{Ho}(Z_{t_1} \geq 2.413$ or $Z_{t_2} \geq 2.413$ or $Z_{t_3} \geq 2.413$ or $Z_{t_4} \geq 2.413$ or $Z_{t_5} \geq 2.413)$
$= \ldots$ (similar steps)
$= 0.0219 + 0.0031$
$= 0.0250$. Thus, $\alpha(t_5 = 1) = 0.0250$

We can graph (0, 0.0079, 0.0138, 0.0183, 0.0219, 0.0250) versus (0, 0.2, 0.4, 0.6, 0.8, 1) to find this cumulative alpha-spending function.

Example 8.3

$K = 5$, $\alpha = 0.025$, OBF boundary: (4.562, 3.223, 2.634, 2.281, 2.040). Following similar steps as done previously, we can obtain the (discrete) type I error spending function $\alpha(t_1 = 1/5) = 0.0000$, $\alpha(t_2 = 2/5) = 0.0006$, $\alpha(t_3 = 3/5) = 0.0045$, $\alpha(t_4 = 4/5) = 0.0128$, and $\alpha(t_5 = 1) = 0.0250$ (Homework 8.2).

8.2.4 Pocock-Type, OBF-Type, and Other Continuous Boundaries

Removing the restriction of a fixed K and equally spaced $t_i = i/K$, Lan and DeMets (1983) gave the continuous alpha-spending function for the general Pocock-type boundary as

$$\alpha_{Pocock}(t) = \alpha \ln [1 + (e - 1)t] \tag{8.5}$$

and for the general OBF-type boundary as

$$\alpha_{OBF}(t) = 2\left[1 - \Phi\left(\frac{z_{\alpha/2}}{\sqrt{t}}\right)\right] \tag{8.6}$$

where $\Phi(.)$ is the cdf of the standard normal distribution.

The boundaries corresponding to the continuous alpha-spending functions are approximately close to the original discrete, equally spaced boundaries. The *x-type boundary* describes the fact that these continuous boundaries differ from, but follow closely, the characteristics of the original Pocock boundary, being flat with constant critical values throughout the study, and that of the original OBF boundary, being very stringent in the beginning of the trial then decreasing as information is gathered.

Other type I error rate continuous spending functions have also been proposed in the literature. Kim and DeMets (1987) studied certain members of the *power family*

$$\alpha(t) = \alpha t^c, \quad c > 0$$

The power $c = 1$ corresponds to the linear or uniform spending (i.e., the Pocock type) and $c = 3$ closely resembles the OBF type.

The landmark clinical trial Scandinavian Simvastatin Survival Study (4S) (1993) (mentioned in Chapter 2) used a member of the *truncated exponential distribution family* of alpha-spending functions proposed by Hwang, Shih, and DeCani (1990):

$$\alpha(\gamma, t) = \alpha\left[\frac{1 - e^{-\gamma t}}{1 - e^{\gamma}}\right], \quad \gamma \neq 0 \quad \text{for } 0 \leq t \leq 1 \tag{8.7}$$

$$= \alpha t, \quad \gamma = 0$$

We can see here that $\gamma = 0$ is the uniform spending, $\gamma > 0$ is the concave spending and $\gamma < 0$ is the convex spending of the type I error rate. Concave spending of alpha is suitable for short-term trials with an immediate response, such as for single dose analgesic studies, where accelerated early stopping is desirable in early phases of drug development; usually $1 \leq \gamma \leq 4$. Convex spending of alpha is suitable for large trials in chronic diseases where patient recruitment is slow and staggered and follow-up is long, so that very early termination with limited samples is not encouraged; usually, $-5 \leq \gamma \leq -1$. For example, the 4S trial used $\gamma = -4$.

The (continuous) Pocock-type boundary is included in Equation 8.7, with $\gamma = 1$; the (continuous) OBF-type boundary is also a member of Equation 8.7, with approximately $\gamma = -4$ or -5; the *power family* member $\alpha(t) = \alpha t^{3/2}$ is closely approximated by $\gamma = -1$, and $\alpha(t) = \alpha t^2$ is approximated by $\gamma = -2$. See Hwang, Shih, and DeCani (1990) for a graph of alpha-spending rate and table of boundaries of this general family of alpha-spending functions.

In-Class Exercise: The calculation of the boundaries requires iterative numerical integrations. SAS and R, as well as some commercial software, are available for obtaining the boundaries. Preference is given to the software provided by the University of Wisconsin, which can be acquired by following the steps provided. A reference for this software is given in Reboussin et al. (2000).

Go to the following University of Wisconsin web page to download the Lan-DeMets software to your computer step by step and perform the practice sessions in this chapter.

- https://www.biostat.wisc.edu/content/lan-demetsmethod-statistical-programsclinical-trials
- Under the heading "Programs for Computing Group Sequential Boundaries Using the Lan-DeMets Method," click on the red Download link for Windows to download WinLD.exe, or download the MSDOS executable ld98.exe. Unzip the file and install.
- The WinLD.chm file is the user manual; it contains some good examples.

Practice 8.1: Run the Lan-DeMets software. Under Compute, select Bounds.

1. Design boundaries (Set up to plan a trial protocol)

    Compute the boundaries of the Pocock and OBF types and the power family with appropriate power parameters to match the Hwang, Shih, and DeCani truncated exponential family with appropriate parameters. Compare them with the discrete, equally spaced Pocock and OBF boundaries in Section 8.2.2 (for K = 5).

For example, the upper two-sided $\alpha = 0.05$ symmetrical, discrete, equally spaced Pocock boundary for $K = 5$ is (2.413, 2.413, 2.413, 2.413, 2.413). In contrast, the Pocock-type boundary based on Equation 8.5 is not exactly as flat as that, but is (2.4380, 2.4268, 2.4101, 2.3966, 2.3859).

2. Updating boundaries when monitoring a trial

Suppose that the trial initially used $K = 5$ with a (continuous) equally spaced OBF-type boundary in the design. Consider the two scenarios:

a. At the first interim analysis, the actual information time turns out to be $t_1 = 0.3$ (as opposed to planned $t_1 = 0.2$), and the trial design is now rescheduled to $t_2 = 0.75$ and $t_3 = 1$ for the next interim and final analyses. Compute the revised OBF-type boundary.

The $K = 5$ equally spaced, upper two-sided $\alpha = 0.05$ symmetrical OBF-type boundary is (4.8769, 3.3569, 2.6803, 2.2898, 2.0310). The revised schedule (0.3, 0.75, 1.0) leads to a different boundary (3.9286, 2.3403, 2.0118).

The second scenario: (ii) After the first interim analysis (at $t_1 = 0.2$), the trial continues, but the schedule of subsequent interim analyses has been changed to $t_2 = 3/5$, followed by the final analysis at $t_3 = 1$. The revised schedule (0.2, 0.6, 1.0) leads to the boundary: (4.8769, 2.6686, 1.9809). It is quite clear that the first critical value (4.8769) remains unchanged as planned, because it has already been used by the first interim analysis at the planned time $t_1 = 0.2$).

In both scenarios, for the subsequent changes of frequency and schedule, we have to make sure that these changes are due to administrative reasons (e.g., the enrollment rate has been slower or faster than expected), not prompted by the interim result of the first analysis. Thus, it is obvious that the DMC needs to be independent from the trial sponsor and that the trial sponsor should not be provided with the interim unblinded data.

8.3 Power, Information, and Drift Parameter

Group sequential methods provide a chance for early termination of a trial by rejecting H_o in such a way that the overall type I error rate is maintained. The trade-off, however, is some loss of power, because the tests at early stages involve smaller sample sizes, and the rejection regions are tighter at later stages; both resulting in lower power. In order to maintain the same power as the fixed-size design, a group sequential trial would require a larger *maximum* information/sample size, but the *average* (expected) information/sample size would be smaller (under H_A). The maximum information/sample size is a function of the type I and type II errors, the number of analyses, and the strategy of spending α (i.e., the boundaries for the interim and final analyses).

- Given $b_1, b_2, \ldots, b_K$ (determined by the alpha-spending strategy),

  Power $= 1 - \beta = P_{HA}$ (Reject H_0) $= P_{HA}$ ($Z_{t_1} \geq b_1$ or $Z_{t_2} \geq b_2$ or $\ldots Z_{t_3} \geq b_K$) as a function of the treatment effect (expressed in terms of the *drift* parameter; see Equation 8.8 below).

- Conversely, given power (by the fixed sample size design), we can calculate N_{max} (or in general, I_{max}) for a group sequential design (specified by the boundary) through the calculation of the *drift* parameter, as explained in the following paragraphs.

It is helpful to start with a fixed sample size and adjust it to obtain the maximum sample size for the sequential design. From the sample size calculation in Equation 4.2 (Chapter 4) for a fixed sample size design (with equal treatment group allocation, n subjects per group), we saw the basic relationship $E(Z) = z_\alpha + z_\beta$, where $Z = \sqrt{\dfrac{n}{2}} \dfrac{\bar{X}_n - \bar{Y}_n}{\sigma}$, and $\varphi_f \equiv E(Z) = \sqrt{\dfrac{n}{2}} \dfrac{\Delta}{\sigma}$, which is the *noncentrality parameter* of the fixed-size z-test under H_A that pivots the power of the test (see Equation 4.5). Note that $\varphi_f^2 \propto n$.

For a sequential design, the interim stage sample size at a given time $t = n/n_{max}$ is $n = n_{max}t$, and the final $N_{max} = 2n_{max}$ is the *maximum* sample size at $t = 1$. The test statistic of the interim analysis, $Z(t)$, is based on the interim sample size n (per group). The sample size of the fixed-size design (without any interim analysis) corresponds to the (final) maximum sample size of the sequential design. Thus,

$$EZ(t) = \sqrt{\frac{n}{2}} \frac{\Delta}{\sigma} = \sqrt{t} \sqrt{\frac{n_{max}}{2}} \frac{\Delta}{\sigma} = \sqrt{t}\varphi \qquad (8.8)$$

where $\varphi \equiv Z(t = 1) = \sqrt{\dfrac{n_{max}}{2}} \dfrac{\Delta}{\sigma}$ is called the *drift* parameter in the Lan-DeMets program for the sequential design. It corresponds to the noncentrality parameter φ_f for the fixed-size design.

Recall that, when using $\bar{X}_n - \bar{Y}_n$ to estimate the treatment mean difference Δ, $Var(\bar{X}_n - \bar{Y}_n) = \dfrac{2\sigma^2}{n}$, $I_n = \dfrac{n}{2\sigma^2}$. Therefore, in a sequential trial, Equation 8.8 can also be written as

$$EZ(t) = \sqrt{\frac{n}{2}} \frac{\Delta}{\sigma} = \sqrt{I_n} \Delta = \sqrt{tI_{max}} \Delta \qquad (8.9)$$

Hence, $$\varphi = EZ(t = 1) = \sqrt{I_{max}} \Delta \qquad (8.10)$$

TABLE 8.2

Drift Parameter of the Score Test

Comparison	Drift Parameter	Note
Normal means	$\sqrt{n_{max}}\sqrt{1/2\sigma^2}(\mu_x - \mu_y)$	n = per group size
Binomial probabilities	$\sqrt{n_{max}}\sqrt{1/2\overline{pq}}(p_x - p_y)$	n = per group size $\overline{p}=(1-\overline{q})=(p_x+p_y)/2$
Survival distributions (log-rank test)	$\sqrt{D_{max}}\sqrt{1/4}\log(HR)$	D = total deaths HR = hazard ratio

Next, we set up the maximum information of a sequential design from the corresponding fixed-size design. We see from Equation 8.10 that $\varphi^2 \propto I_{max}$. Without interim analyses, recall that for $Z \sim N(E(Z), 1)$, $\varphi_f \equiv E(Z) = z_\alpha + z_\beta$ is the drift parameter for the fixed-size design. For example, $\alpha = 0.025$, $1 - \beta = 0.90$, implying that $\varphi_f = 1.96 + 1.28 = 3.24$. With K = 5 equally spaced interim analyses, using the OBF-type boundary, we get $\varphi = 3.2788$ from the Lan-DeMets program. Therefore, $(\varphi/\varphi_f)^2 = (3.2788/3.24)^2 = 1.024$. The maximum information of a sequential design requires 1.024 times the corresponding information of the fixed-size design. The size inflation of 2.4% may not be a lot for a small study, but it may mean a lot for a large trial. In general, for boundaries such as those of the OBF type, when the final critical value is close to $z_{\alpha/2}$, the sample size inflation factor is not large. For the Pocock-type boundary, it can be substantial. However, in all cases, the expected information required for a sequential trial would be less than the fixed-size design due to the possibility of early termination.

The drift parameters derived from the score (asymptotic) z-tests for comparing two normal means, two binomial probabilities, and two survival distributions (with the log-rank test) are listed in Table 8.2.

In-Class Exercise

Practice 8.2: For two-sided $\alpha = 0.05$, $1 - \beta = 0.90$, with K = 5 equally spaced interim analyses, using the OBF-type boundary, use the Lan-DeMets program (via Compute Drift) to calculate the drift parameter to get $\varphi = 3.2788$ and calculate the sample size inflation factor.

8.4 P-Value When Trial Is Stopped

At each time t, we calculate the z-statistic, z(t) and the predefined boundary. When the test statistic crosses the boundary, we have the stopping time (τ). When we observe (t, z(τ)) and stop the trial, we need to report the *p-value*. The p-value is the probability under the null of obtaining a result that is at least as extreme as the observed one, that is (t, z(τ)). Therefore, we need to incorporate *order* for the two-dimensional summary statistic (t, z(t)).

There are different ways of ordering in this two-dimensional space. The most commonly one used is the following *stage-wise ordering*:

$$(\tau_2, z(\tau_2)) \prec (\tau_1, z(\tau_1)) \text{ if and only if } \tau_2 < \tau_1 \text{ or when } \tau_2 = \tau_1, z(\tau_2) \geq \tau_1 z(\tau_1) \qquad (8.11)$$

That is, we compare the stopping time first. An earlier stopping time is more extreme than a later stopping time. With the same stopping time, then a larger test statistic is more extreme. Hence, with the stage-wise ordering, for outcome $(\tau = t_j, Z(t_j) = z_j)$, more extreme outcomes are those pairs that either have the test statistic crossing the boundary at an earlier time $t = 1, \ldots, j-1$, or stops at $t = j$ but with a larger statistic than the observed z_j. Thus, the p-value is calculated by the following probability under the null hypothesis

$$p = Pr\left(\bigcup_{i=1}^{j-1} Z(t_i) \geq b_i \cup Z(t_j) \geq z_j \right) \qquad (8.12)$$

We can see that the interim analysis adjusted p-value only depends on boundaries before and at the stopping time, not after. (When using the Lan-DeMets program, one may put arbitrary boundaries after j, as the calculation of the cumulative exit probability will only be up to j.) The adjusted p-value in Equation 8.12 is approximately equal to the unadjusted p-value $Pr(Z(t_j) \geq z_j)$ for large b_i, $i < j$. Large boundary values make early stopping more difficult, hence the adjustment of the p-value is negligible. For example, for the OBF-type boundaries, the adjusted p-value is close to the unadjusted p-value.

In-Class Exercise
Practice 8.3: We are monitoring a trial that is designed with five equally spaced interim analyses by the OBF-type boundary z-values: 4.88, 3.36, 2.68, 2.29, 2.03. After observing (0.6, Z(0.6) = 2.94), since 2.94 > 2.68, the trial stops with t = 0.6. The p-value = $Pr(Z(0.2) \geq 4.88$ or $Z(0.4) \geq 3.36$ or $Z(0.6) \geq 2.94) = 0.00183$ by numerical integration. Note that the unadjusted $Pr(Z \geq 2.94) = 0.00164$.

In the Lan-DeMets program, select Compute Probabilities and User Input to specify the boundaries. Input boundaries $(b_1, b_2, \ldots, b_{j-1}, z_j) = (4.88, 3.36, 2.94)$ and arbitrary boundaries after 2.94. After clicking Calculate, read the *cumulative exit probabilities* up to $\tau = 0.6$.

8.5 Estimation of Treatment Effect

Not only do we need to report the p-value, we often also need to estimate the treatment effect after the trial stops. The drift parameter (see Table 8.2) is also used for estimating the (standardized) treatment effect after we observe (τ_{obs}, z_{obs}). For example, for the difference of means, we calculate the $100(1-\alpha)\%$ confidence interval (ϕ_L, ϕ_U) from

$$P_{\phi_L}\{(\tau, Z(\tau)) \succ (\tau_{obs}, z_{obs})\} = \alpha/2$$

and
$$P_{\phi_U}\{(\tau, Z(\tau)) \prec (\tau_{obs}, z_{obs})\} = \alpha/2$$

Then, convert (ϕ_L, ϕ_U) to the treatment effect via the relationship $\phi = \sqrt{n_{max}} \sqrt{1/2\sigma^2} (\mu_x - \mu_y)$. Other scenarios are given in Table 8.2.

In-Class Exercise
Practice 8.4: This comes from the help manual (WinLD.chm) of the Lan-DeMets program.

Select "Compute Confidence"; Set K = 6, Information times: 0.23, 0.33, 0.44, 0.58, 0.71, 0.83. (User Input the information times. Notice that the last time point is not necessarily 1.)

Specify two-sided symmetric bounds by using the linear spending function (with Function: Power family with Phi = 1)
Standardized Statistic: z = 2.82
Confidence Level: 0.95
Calculate: (ϕ_L, ϕ_U) = (0.19, 4.94) and the boundary

- Convert to CI of (μ_x, μ_y) with the values of n, σ
- Convert to CI of $p_x - p_y$ with the values of n, $\bar{p}$
- Convert to CI of log(HR) with the value of D

The upper bounds are displayed: 2.527, 2.616, 2.562, 2.473, 2.426, 2.388. (Note that the boundary has a hump at the second time point). Because z = 2.82, this indicates that the study would be stopped at the first interim analysis where t = 0.23.

Practice 8.5: The study in Proschan, Lan, and Wittes (2006, 129) is summarized as follows:

- Weight change (kg) over 3 months in n = 200 (per arm).
- Planned K = 4, equal intervals, with the OBF-type boundary.
- Actual t_1 = 0.22, t_2 = 0.55 (not 0.25, 0.5 as planned).
- At the third look, the mean weight loss in the two groups are $\bar{x}_{152}$ = 8.1 kg and $\bar{y}_{144}$ = 6.0 kg (subscript indicates sample size on which the sample mean is based).
- Hence, t_3 = (152 + 144)/400 ≈ 0.74.

- The pooled sd = 4.8 kg, so z = 3.76.
- We want to report the p-value and 95% CI of $\mu_x - \mu_y$.

Answer: Use the Lan-DeMets program to perform the following steps:

1. For p-value: Select Compute Probability
   - K = 4, user input t: 0.22, 0.55, 0.74, 1
   - Two-sided symmetric, OBF spending function ($\alpha = 0.05$)
   - Calculate to get boundaries at t_1 (4.64) and t_2 (2.81)
   - Change Determine Bounds to User Input and fill in the following:
     4.64, 2.81, 3.76 (= z), 1 (arbitrary)
   - Calculate to obtain exit probability = 0.005 (two-sided p-value)
     Note: The unadjusted p-value is $\Pr(|Z| > 3.76) = 0.0002$
2. For CI: Select Compute Confidence Interval
   - K = 4, user input t: 0.22, 0.55, 0.74, 1
   - Two-sided symmetric, change Determine Bounds to User Input and fill in the following:
     4.64, 2.81, 3.76 (= z), 1 (arbitrary)
   - Standardized statistic: 3.76
   - Confidence level: 0.95
   - Calculate to obtain $(\varphi_L, \varphi_U) = (1.106, 5.536)$
   - Convert to CI for $\mu_x - \mu_y$ with n = 200, σ = pooled sd = 4.8 by using

$$\varphi = \sqrt{n_{max}/2\sigma^2}\,(\mu_x - \mu_y)$$

to get $(\Delta_L, \Delta_U) = (0.531, 2.657)$.

Appendix 8.1: R Function *qfind* for Calculating the Critical Value (Boundary) of the Second (Final) Analysis

This function is suitable for a two-stage design with any spending of alpha <0.05 at the first (interim) stage, at any information time <1. No specification of an alpha-spending function is required.

Assumptions include: overall alpha = 0.05, two-sided, symmetric boundaries.

First, install package 'mvtnorm'

```
>library(mvtnorm)
# Input: p1 = interim alpha spent, p2 = 0.05-p1; tfrac =
interim information fraction
# return: (c1, c2) = critical values of the two stages; alpha2
= nominal alpha for c2
qfind <-
function(p1 = 0.01, p2 = 0.04, tfrac = 0.5, tol = 1e-10)
{
        c1 <- qnorm(1 - p1/2)
        low <- 0
        upp <- 4
        mid <- (low + upp)/2
        val <- pbvn(c1, mid, tfrac)
while(abs(val - p2) > tol) {
if(val > p2)
low <- mid
else upp <- mid
mid <- (low + upp)/2
val <- pbvn(c1, mid, tfrac)
}
a2 <- 2 * pnorm(- mid)
out <- c(c1, mid, a2, val)
names(out) <- c("c1", "c2", "alpha2", "p2")
return(out)
}
pbvn <- function(x, y, tfrac = 0.5)
{
2*(pmvnorm(c(-x,-Inf), c(x,-y), corr = matrix(c(1,sqrt(tfrac),
    sqrt(tfrac),1),nrow = 2))[[1]])
}
# Try the default
qfind()
# Example - find the two-sided critical values from a one-
    sided alpha spent
>p1 = 0.002578977
>qfind(p1 = 0.002578977*2,p2 = (0.025-p1)*2,tfrac = 0.5)
```

Appendix 8.2: A Further Note on the Partial Sum Process with Independent Increments

For immediate responses, either continuous or binary, cumulative sums of the independent random variables from time to time are easily seen to have independent increments. The usefulness of this "partial sum with independent increments" property was illustrated in Section 8.2.3. An important development was made by Tsiatis (1981, 1982), who showed that the log-rank statistic computed over time behaves like a partial sum of independent normal random variables. This result extended the use of group sequential methods to clinical trials with survival data. Jennison and Turnbull (1997) provided a unified theory that explains the "independent increments" structure commonly seen in group sequential test statistics. Scharfstein, Tsiatis, and Robbins (1997) demonstrated that all sequentially computed Wald statistics based on efficient estimators, for example, MLEs of the parameter of interest, will under mild regularity conditions have the asymptotic multivariate normal distribution similar to the earlier setup. Hence, the group sequential procedure extends to more complicated situations such as the proportional hazards model (Sellke and Siegmund 1983) and correlated observations including longitudinal data with random effects model (Wei, Su, and Lachin 1990; Lee and DeMets 1991) or with distribution-free analyses (Lachin 1997).

Appendix 8.3: Information Time/Fraction and Maximum-Duration Trial versus Maximum-Information Trial

Taking statistical information as the inverse of the variance of the parameter estimate, Lan and Zucker (1993) defined the *information time/fraction* as the amount of information accrued by calendar time divided by the total information at the scheduled end of the trial. We have seen that the information time played an essential role in the type I error spending-function approach. Depending on the statistics used (Lan, Reboussin, and DeMets 1994), a whole unit information can be approximated by either a subject (for comparing means) or an event (for comparing survival distributions). In either case, the total information must be known. If not known, as is often the case, then the information time/fraction can only be estimated. For example, in the time-to-event case, Tsiatis (1981) showed that the variance of the log-rank statistics, when calculated over time, grows proportionally to the number of events observed. Hence the information time is equal to the proportion of the maximum number of events expected by the end of a study, with the numerator being the observed number of events at the (calendar) time of interim analysis. For a maximum-information trial, the maximum number of events expected by the end of a study is chosen in advance to achieve a desired power, given other design parameters. However, for a maximum-duration trial, that is, when the maximum trial duration is fixed, the maximum information is random. In such a trial, the denominator of the information time can be estimated under either the null or the alternative hypothesis, thus leading to two information timescales.

A natural compromise to overcome this difficulty of uncertain information timescale is to first choose an estimate of the maximum information, either "under the null" or "under the alternative" hypothesis. Then set the information time to be 1 if the proportion exceeds 1 or if the current analysis is the last analysis and the proportion has not yet reached 1. The consequence of this compromise is that the type I error spending function will be altered from the original one that was prespecified in the design. A simple example that illustrates this can be found in Kim, Boucher, and Tsiatis (1995). In real applications, we can only hope that the alpha-spending function will not be altered as much as in this illustrative example.

Example 8.4: Over-Running and Under-Running Change the Alpha-Spending Function

Suppose K = 2 analyses were planned for a trial where the one-sided significance level of 0.05 was specified in the protocol. At the design stage, the uniform (linear) type I error spending function, $\alpha(t) = 0.05t$ was chosen for monitoring. The expected total number of events is 200 under the null hypothesis, but is 100 under the alternative (Figure 8.4). Suppose that there are 50 events at the first analysis. If we have chosen the information timescale based on the null hypothesis, then $t_1 = 50/200 = 0.25$, and $\alpha(t_1) = 0.0125$. The group sequential boundary b_1 such that $P\{Z_{t1} \geq b_1\} = 0.0125$ is $b_1 = 2.24$. Suppose at the final analysis, the number of events is truly 200, as expected under the null hypothesis, the correlation between Z_{t1} and Z_{t2} is $(t_1/t_2)^{1/2} = (0.25)^{1/2} = 0.5$. Thus, the group sequential boundary b_2 such that $P\{Z_{t1} < 2.24, Z_{t2} \geq b_2\} = 0.05 - 0.0125 = 0.0375$ is $b_2 = 1.74$.

However, if the realized number of events at the final analysis turns out to be 100 instead (i.e., an under-running situation), then the "true" t_1 should be $50/100 = 0.5$ and we should have spent $\alpha(t_1) = 0.025$. But we cannot go back in time, because we have already adopted $b_1 = 2.24$ for the test at the first analysis. What we can do is to recognize that (a) at $t_1 = 0.5$ (not 0.25), we used $\alpha(t_1) = 0.0125$ and (b) the correlation

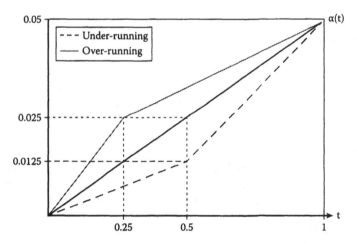

FIGURE 8.4
The alpha-spending function is altered when under-running or over-running of a trial occurs.

between Z_{t1} and Z_{t2} is $(t_1/t_2)^{1/2} = (0.5)^{1/2}$. Thus, the group sequential boundary b_2 such that $P\{Z_{t1} < 2.24, Z_{t2} \geq b_2\} = 0.0375$ is $b_2 = 1.70$. From the fact that $\alpha(0.5) = 0.0125 < 0.025$, we see that the type I error spending function was no longer the uniform (linear) spending-function. Instead, it is a convex function, running under the uniform (linear) spending function.

The over-running case is the opposite, when 100 events under the alternative hypothesis were used to estimate t_1, but 200 events occurred at the final analysis. The consequence is that the linear spending function is altered to a concave function, running over the uniform (linear) spending function.

Homework 8.1

Read the article "Sorafenib in Advanced Hepatocellular Carcinoma" (Llovet, J. M., et al., *New England Journal of Medicine*, 2008, 359(4): 378–390) and identify the trial organization and study monitoring schedules.

Homework 8.2

Work out the steps of constructing the alpha-spending function for the equally spaced $K = 5$ OBF boundary and plot it against the alpha-spending function of the Pocock boundary.

Homework 8.3

For the article "Sorafenib in Advanced Hepatocellular Carcinoma" (Llovet, J. M., et al., *New England Journal of Medicine*, 2008, 359(4): 378–390), do the following:

1. Describe the study design and endpoints of the trial.

2. Determine approximately how much alpha was "spent" at each analysis (two interim and one final) for each endpoint. (Note: The proportion of information at any particular time can be assumed to be roughly approximated by the number of deaths that occurred out of what was expected.)

3. Compare your answer from part (b) to the amount of the type I error that would have been "spent" if a Pocock boundary had been assumed.

4. Give a very brief summary of the results including the stopping decision.

5. Based on Figure 2 of this paper:

   a. Compare between treatments with respect to the 25th, 50th, and 75th percentiles for each endpoint.

   b. Compare across treatments with respect to the probability of survival, the probability of symptomatic progression, and the probability of radiologic progression at 9 months.

References

Armitage P, McPherson CK, and Rowe BC. (1969). Repeated significance tests on accumulating data. *Journal of the Royal Statistical Society, Series A* 132: 235–244.

DeMets DL and Ware JH. (1982). Asymmetric group sequential boundaries for monitoring clinical trials. *Biometrika* 69: 661–663.

Ellenberg SS. (2001). Independent data monitoring committees: rationale, operations and controversies. *Statistics in Medicine* 20: 2573–2583.

FDA (US Department of Health and Human Services, Food and Drug Administration). (2006). *Guidance for Clinical Trial Sponsors: Establishment and Operation of Clinical Trial Data Monitoring Committees.* http://www.fda.gov/AboutFDA/CentersOffices/OfficeofMedicalProductsandTobacco/CDER/ManualofPoliciesProcedures/ (accessed on 2/17/2014).

Haybittle JL. (1971). Repeated assessment of results in clinical trials of cancer treatment. *British Journal of Radiology* 44: 793–797.

Hwang IK, Shih WJ, and DeCani JS. (1990). Group sequential designs using a family of Type I error probability spending functions. *Statistics in Medicine* 9: 1439–1445.

ICH (International Conference on Harmonisation of Technical Requirements for Registration of Pharmaceuticals for Human Use). (1996). *Guideline for Industry: E3 Structure and Content of Clinical Study Reports.* http://www.fda.gov/downloads/drugs/guidancecomplianceregulatoryinformation/guidances/ucm073113.pdf (accessed on 4/20/2015).

ICH. (1998). *Guidance for Industry: E9 Statistical Principles for Clinical Trials.* http://www.fda.gov/downloads/drugs/guidancecomplianceregulatoryinformation/guidances/ucm073137.pdf (accessed on 2/17/2014).

Jennison C and Turnbull BW. (1997). Group-sequential analysis incorporating covariate information. *Journal of the American Statistical Association* 92: 1330–1341.

Kim KM and DeMets DL. (1987). Design and analysis of group sequential tests based on Type I error spending rate function. *Biometrika* 74: 149–154.

Kim KM, Boucher H, and Tsiatis AA. (1995). Design and analysis of group sequential Logrank tests in maximum duration versus information trials. *Biometrics* 51: 988–1000.

Lachin JM (1997). Group sequential monitoring of distribution-free analyses of repeated measures. *Statistics in Medicine* 16: 653–668.

Lan KKG and DeMets DL. (1983). Discrete sequential boundaries for clinical trials. *Biometrika* 70: 659–663.

Lan KKG and Wittes J. (1988). The B-value: a tool for monitoring data. *Biometrics* 44: 579–585.

Lan KKG and Zucker D. (1993). Sequential monitoring for clinical trials: the role of information and Brownian motion. *Statistics in Medicine* 12: 753–765.

Lan KKG, Reboussin DM, and DeMets DL. (1994). Information and information fractions for designing sequential monitoring of clinical trials. *Communications in Statistics (A)—Theory and Methods* 23: 403–420.

Lee JW and DeMets DL. (1991). Sequential comparison of changes with repeated measurements data. *Journal of American Statistical Association* 86: 757–762.

Llovet JM, Ricci S, Mazzaferro V, Hilgard P, Gane E, Blanc JF, de Oliveira AC et al. The SHARP Investigators Study Group. (2008). Sorafenib in advanced Hepatocellular Carcinoma. *New England Journal of Medicine* 359: 378–390.

O'Brien PC and Fleming TR. (1979). A multiple testing procedure for clinical trials. *Biometrics* 35: 549–556.

Peto R, Pike MC, Armitage P, Breslow NE, Cox DR, Howard SV, Mantel N, et al. (1976). Design and analysis of randomized clinical trials requiring prolonged observation of each patient. *British Journal of Cancer* 35: 585–611.

Pocock SJ. (1977). Group sequential methods in the design and analysis of clinical trials. *Biometrika* 64: 191–199.

Proschan MA, Lan KKG, and Wittes JT. (2006). *Statistical Monitoring of Clinical Trials: A Unified Approach*. New York: Springer.

Reboussin DM, DeMets DL, Kim KM, and Lan KKG. (2000). Computations for group sequential boundaries using the Lan-DeMets spending function method. *Controlled Clinical Trials* 21: 190–207.

Scandinavian Simvastatin Survival Study Group. (1993). Design and baseline results of the Scandinavian Simvastatin survival study of patients with stable Angina and/ or previous myocardial infarction. *The American Journal of Cardiology* 71: 393–400.

Scharfstein DO, Tsiatis AA, and Robbins JM. (1997). Semiparametric efficiency and its implication on the design and analysis of group sequential studies. *Journal of the American Statistical Association* 92: 1342–1350.

Sellke T and Siegmund D. (1983). Sequential analysis of the proportional hazards model. *Biometrika* 70: 315–326.

Shih WJ. (2000). Group sequential methods. In *Encyclopedia of Biopharmaceutical Statistics*, Chow SC (Ed.), New York: Marcel-Dekker.

Slud ER and Wei LJ. (1982). Two-sample repeated significance tests based on the modified Wilcoxon statistic. *Journal of the American Statistical Association* 77: 862–868.

Tsiatis AA. (1981). The asymptotic joint distribution of the efficient scores test for the proportional hazards model calculated over time. *Biometrika* 68: 311–315.

Tsiatis AA. (1982). Repeated significance testing for a general class of statistics used in censored survival analysis. *Journal of the American Statistical Association* 77: 855–861.

Wei LJ, Su JQ, and Lachin JM. (1990). Interim analyses with repeated measurements in a sequential clinical trial. *Biometrika* 77: 359–364.

9

Monitoring the Maximum Information

In previous chapters, we discussed the fixed-size design without interim analysis, as well as sequential designs with interim analyses. The alpha-spending function approach of the classical group sequential (GS) design is particularly useful in providing a flexible tool for monitoring the safety and efficacy aspects of clinical trials. In particular, this approach provides flexibility in the schedule and the number of interim analyses. The fundamental structure of the fixed-size design without interim analyses and the classical GS procedure with interim analyses relies on maximum, fixed, and prespecified information in the study protocol. The information times (fractions) used for interim analyses are based on this fixed, prespecified, maximum information. What if the prespecified maximum information is incorrect? Can it be altered later if it is found to be inadequate? These questions are often asked. Recall that in Chapter 4 we discussed how sample size calculation, study power, and values for design parameters such as treatment effect, within-group variance, compliance rate, etc., had to be assumed, ideally based on data derived from prior studies with very similar design conditions, especially for Phase III confirmatory studies. However, we often find that the prior studies, if any, usually involve different patient populations (defined by the inclusion and exclusion criteria and different staging technologies), medical practices (e.g., allowable concomitant medications), study durations, or treatment regimens. An intriguing idea, therefore, would be to see if these assumptions could be verified or updated with interim data from the ongoing study. For example, after checking the interim data, we find that an extension of the (initial) maximum information is necessary to ensure the study power. With this finding, we would then need to modify the original sample size and perhaps also the conventional fixed-size test or the classical sequential procedure. In performing all these modifications, we would then need to ensure that the type I error rate remained protected. A recent development in this area is termed *adaptive designs* or *flexible designs*. In this chapter, we discuss three topics related to the adaptive or flexible designs: (i) sample size reestimation (SSR) with continuous or binary endpoints, (ii) monitoring trial duration for maximum information (for event-driven trials) or maximum duration (for duration driven trials) with survival endpoints, and (iii) modification of the classical GS alpha-spending function. In both SSR and monitoring trial duration, the methods involve only blinded data. For the modification of the alpha-spending function, we use unblinded interim data. SSR and monitoring trial duration with unblinded data remains an ongoing research topic and is beyond the scope of this book. Overall, the recent development of adaptive designs offers trials great flexibility in making midcourse modifications of the maximum information or duration, but there could be some potential pitfalls. Examples are given to illustrate some vigilant points.

9.1 Sample Size Reestimation

In order to protect the integrity of an ongoing trial, the blindness of the study is best kept intact. A simple method for SSR would be to check the total variance for trials using a continuous primary endpoint or to check the pooled event rate for trials using a binary primary endpoint, based on the blind interim data. If the total variance or pooled event rate is found higher or lower than expected, respectively, compared to the original assumptions, then we increase the sample size to achieve the desired study power. Otherwise, the study continues with the original sample size. SSR using blind interim data without the possibility of downsizing will not change the type I error rate, because the variance and pooled event rate are the nuisance parameters (parameters that are separated from the treatment difference, delta). The power and SSR still remain based on the treatment effect (delta) that the protocol authors assumed in the original alternative hypothesis. Because increasing the sample size of an ongoing trial involves many administrative and logistical matters and possibly delaying the trial, we usually perform SSR only once in the course of a study. The timing of when we perform an SSR also needs attention. We need enough data to make the interim analysis reliable. On the other hand, the later the interim analysis, the harder we find it to make administrative changes to the trial, such as amending the protocol, going through IRBs, selecting new medical centers, contracting new investigators, enrolling more patients, etc.

More sophisticated methods for SSR are available. For example, we can use the EM (expectation-maximization) algorithm for solving a mixture of two normal distributions with a common variance (see Shih 1992; Gould and Shih 1992), which is based on the idea that the unavailable treatment group identification is "missing completely at random" (MCAR)—see Chapter 10 for the topic of missing data. However, most of the practitioners prefer the above simple methods (i.e., just using the total variance). If, however, concern remains that the total variance may be too large compared to the within-group variance used in the original sample size calculation, one may consider using a correction formula that involves assumed treatment difference, delta, as follows:

Let S_T^2 be the sample estimate of the total variance, and S_W^2 be the (pooled) estimate of the within-group variance. We can show that

$$(2n_1 - 1)S_T^2 = n_1 \hat{\Delta}^2/2 + 2(n_1 - 1)S_W^2 \tag{9.1}$$

The proof may be done for homework (Homework 9.1). Note that in the ANOVA setting the left side of Equation 9.1 is the "corrected total of sum of squares," the second term of the right side is the "within-group sum of squares," and the multipliers involving the per-group sample size n_1 are the corresponding degrees of freedom. Of course, because of the blinding, neither the estimate of the treatment effect, $\hat{\Delta}$, nor the estimate of the within-group variance, S_W^2, are actually observed. Gould and Shih (1992) suggested the use of the original hypothesized Δ_0 to replace $\hat{\Delta}$ in Equation 9.1 and then obtained the following estimate of the pseudo-within-group variance:

$$S^2 = \left[(2n_1 - 1)S_T^2 - n_1\Delta_0^2/2\right]/2(n_1 - 1) \tag{9.2}$$

An alternative correction strategy uses the mean squared error of a regression model with some baseline covariate other than the (unavailable) treatment group. Of course in either correction we never know whether the adjustment will be enough or inadequate, depending on the assumed delta, for the first way of correction, and the correlation of the covariate with the response, for the second way of correction, relative to the true treatment effect.

Proschan, Lan, and Wittes (2006) pointed out that based on Equation 9.1 the ratio of the total variance to the within-group variance can be expressed as

$$\frac{S_T^2}{S_W^2} = \frac{n_1\hat{\Delta}^2}{2(2n_1 - 1)S_W^2} + \frac{2(n_1 - 1)}{2n_1 - 1} \approx 1 + \frac{1}{4}\left(\frac{\hat{\Delta}}{S_W}\right)^2$$

The effect size $\dfrac{\hat{\Delta}}{S_W}$ in a typical Phase III trial is around 0.2 to 0.5 (see Section 4.2). This gives us some idea of the range of the inflation when we use the total variance estimate instead of the (unobserved) within-group variance estimate.

9.2 Monitoring Trial Duration for Studies with Survival Endpoints

Clinical trials with survival endpoints usually require a long duration in order to enroll enough patients and incur enough events. When we specify maximum information (i.e., the total number of events) in the protocol for a desirable study power, the length of the trial then becomes random. Although we specify the projected length of the study at the beginning of the trial, we believe it prudent, and in fact a common practice, for the sponsor of such a resource-demanding trial to reestimate the end time of the trial based on interim data during the trial's progress. Below is an example to illustrate this point.

Example 9.1

A trial is designed to require 120 primary events with a plan to enroll 230 patients. Eighteen months after randomizing the first patient, an interim analysis with blinded data reveals a total of 111 enrolled subjects and shows the following information: total patient exposure time of 65 patient-years, 16 primary events out of the 111 enrolled subjects, and 10 subjects who dropped out early (lost to follow-up) without a primary event before withdrawal.

Using simple or crude estimates, we calculate the rate of subject recruitment at about $111/18 = 6$ patients per month, the event rate at $16/65 = 0.25$ events per patient-year, and the patient early withdrawal rate at $10/65 = 0.15$ withdraws per patient-year. The question we then pose is: If the trial continued at the same enrollment rate, withdrawal rate, and event rate, how long would it take for the study to reach the full 120 events?

We first derive the general solution, then come back to this specific example.

Let T_j be the potential event time and U_j the censoring time of subject j. The variable T_j will be observed whenever $T_j \leq U_j$. Let $X_j = \min(T_j, U_j)$, and $\delta_j = I_{\{T_j \leq U_j\}}$, where I_A is the indicator function for event A. The data is the set $\{X_j, \delta_j, j = 1, \ldots, n\}$ and the counting process as a function of time t is $N_j(t) = I_{\{X_j \leq t, \delta_j = 1\}}$. Then, we derive

$$E\, N_j(t) = \Pr(X_j \leq t, \delta_j = 1) = \Pr(T_j \leq t, T_j \leq U_j)$$

$$= \Pr(\text{subject } j \text{ will have event by time } t, \text{ from time } 0)$$
$$(\text{i.e., observation period is } t)$$

$$= E_T\, \Pr(T_j \leq t, T_j \leq U_j | T_j)$$

Assuming T and U are independent, we find that

$$EN_j(t) = \int_0^t H(s)f(s)\,ds \tag{9.3}$$

where $H(s) = \Pr(U > s)$, and f is the density of T.

The above censoring mechanism U may be a competing risk to the primary event, including dropout (i.e., loss to follow-up), or administrative censoring due to staggered entry and data review at time t. The origin of time $(t = 0)$ is the study start (first patient randomization) day.

For example, suppose that the primary event and censoring are independent with exponential distributions: $H(s) = Pr(U > s) = e^{-\eta s}$, $f(s) = \lambda e^{-\lambda s}$. Then following Equation 9.3,

Pr(subject j will have event by time t)

$$
= \int_0^t H(s)f(s)ds = \int_0^t e^{-\eta s}\lambda e^{-\lambda s}ds = \lambda \int_0^t e^{-(\eta+\lambda)s}ds
$$

$$
(9.4)
$$

$$
= \frac{\lambda}{(\eta+\lambda)} \int_0^t (\eta+\lambda)e^{-(\eta+\lambda)s}ds = \frac{\lambda}{(\eta+\lambda)}\left[1-e^{-(\eta+\lambda)t}\right]
$$

We saw this formula previously in Chapter 4 for sample size calculation and continue to use this convenient exponential model to monitor the study progress.

Let n be the total number of subjects planned to be enrolled in the study, and n_1 be the number of subjects enrolled at the interim analysis time t_1 ($n = 230$, $n_1 = 111$, $t_1 = 18$ months in the above example). Suppose that, when we reviewed the data at time t_1, we found d_1 events and r dropouts. Hence, (n_1-d_1-r) subjects remain to be followed-up until the final analysis time, t_2. We call these n_1-d_1-r patients Cohort Q_a.

For Cohort Q_a,
Pr(subject j in these (n_1-d_1-r) will have an event by time t_2, *from time t_1*)

$$
\int_{t_1}^{t_2} H(s)f(s)ds = \frac{\lambda}{(\eta+\lambda)}\left[1-e^{-(\eta+\lambda)(t_2-t_1)}\right]
$$

$$
(9.5)
$$

(observation period is t_2-t_1)

The expected number of events by time t_2 in the patients of Cohort Q_a then is

$$
E_a = (n_1 - d - r)\frac{\lambda}{(\eta+\lambda)}\left[1-e^{-(\eta+\lambda)(t_2-t_1)}\right]
$$

$$
(9.6)
$$

Furthermore, when we review the data at time t_1, another $n_2 = n - n_1$ future subjects are to be enrolled between the time interval (t_1, t_R) and followed-up until t_2 (the final analysis time). We call these n_2 subjects Cohort Q_b.

For Cohort Q_b, we need to include the patient entry time distribution into Equation 9.3. Let y_j be subject j's entry time. Y has the density function g(y) for $t_1 \le y \le t_R$. Let T_j be the potential event time and U_j be the censoring time of subject j; both are relative to the entry time y_j, and all are mutually independent. At calendar/real time t (relative to the study start time 0), the patient's study duration is $t-y_j$. We count subject j as having an event at time t only when the event happens within his or her study duration,

$T_j \le (t-y_j)$, *and* happens before he/she drops out, $T_j \le U_j$; that is, the variable T_j will be observed whenever $T_j \le \min((t-y_j), U_j)$. Let $X_j(t) = \min(T_j, U_j, t-y_j)$, and $\delta_j = I_{\{T_j \le \min(t-y_j, U_j)\}}$, the data is the set $\{X_j, \delta_j, j = 1, \ldots, n\}$ as before, and the counting process as a function of time t is $N_j(t) = I_{\{X_j \le t, \delta_j = 1\}}$.

For Cohort Q_b, the observation period length is t_2-t_1; the cumulative event rate at time $t_2 \ge t_R$ is

$$E\, N_j(t_2) = Pr(X_j \le t_2, \delta_j = 1)$$

$$= Pr(\text{subject } j \text{ will have event by time } t_2, \textit{from time } t_1)$$

$$= E_y\, Pr(T_j \le t_2, T_j \le U_j, T_j \le (t_2-y_j)|y_j)$$

$$= E_y\, Pr(T_j \le U_j, T_j \le (t_2-y_j)|y_j)$$

Y, T, U are mutually independent, and from Equation 9.3

$$= \int_{t_1}^{t_R} \left[\int_0^{t_2-y} H(s)f(s)ds \right] g(y)dy \tag{9.7}$$

For example, with the exponential model as before, $H(s) = Pr(U > s) = e^{-\eta s}$, $f(s) = \lambda e^{-\lambda s}$, and with uniform entry pattern between $t_1 \le y \le t_R$, $g(y) = 1/(t_R-t_1)$. Equation 9.7 indicates that

Pr(subject j in Cohort Q_b will have event by time t_2, *from time t_1*)

$$= \int_{t_1}^{t_R} \left[\int_0^{t_2-y} H(s)f(s)ds \right] g(y)dy$$

$$= \frac{1}{t_R-t_1} \int_{t_1}^{t_R} \left[\int_0^{t_2-y} H(s)f(s)ds \right] dy$$

$$= \frac{1}{t_R-t_1} \int_{t_1}^{t_R} \frac{\lambda}{(\eta+\lambda)} \left[1-e^{-(\eta+\lambda)(t_2-y)} \right] dy$$

$$= \frac{\lambda}{(\eta+\lambda)} \left[1-\left(\frac{1}{(\eta+\lambda)(t_R-t_1)} \right)\left(e^{-(\eta+\lambda)(t_2-t_R)} - e^{-(\eta+\lambda)(t_2-t_1)} \right) \right]$$

The expected number of events by time t_2 in the patients of Cohort Q_b is

$$E_b = (n-n_1)\frac{\lambda}{(\eta+\lambda)} \left[1-\left(\frac{1}{(\eta+\lambda)(t_R-t_1)} \right)\left(e^{-(\eta+\lambda)(t_2-t_R)} - e^{-(\eta+\lambda)(t_2-t_1)} \right) \right] \tag{9.8}$$

Therefore, the additional total number of events expected at time t_2 is $d_2 = E_a + E_b$, the sum of Equations 9.6 and 9.8.

Given a fixed total information (event-driven trials) $E_T = d_1 + d_2$, we can solve for t_2 to answer the question: How long will it take for the study to reach the full number of required events?

On the other hand, for a maximum duration trial (t_2 is fixed) to reach a certain number of events determined by power, we can solve for the required number of patients, n.

For either question, the parameters η and λ are plugged in by their estimates from the interim data. For Example 9.1, which is an event-driven trial, the required total number of events to reach is $120 = d_1 + d_2$. At the interim analysis, we have $n_1 = 111$, $n - n_1 = 230 - 111 = 119$, $d_1 = 16$, $r = 10$, $\lambda = 16/(65*12)$, $\eta = 10/(65*12)$, $t_1 = 18$. Assuming the trial continues with the same uniform enrollment rate ($111/18 \approx 6$ patients per month), then $t_R = 18 + (119/6) \approx 38$ months. If we assume a more conservative uniform enrollment rate of 5 patients per month, then $t_R = 18 + (119/5) \approx 42$ months.

Therefore, we plug in the above information from the interim data in the following equation and solve for t_2:

$$120 - d_1 = (n_1 - d_1 - r)\frac{\lambda}{(\eta + \lambda)}\left[1 - e^{-(\eta + \lambda)(t_2 - t_1)}\right]$$
$$+ (n - n_1)\frac{\lambda}{(\eta + \lambda)}\left[1 - \left(\frac{1}{(\eta + \lambda)(t_R - t_1)}\right)\left(e^{-(\eta + \lambda)(t_2 - t_R)} - e^{-(\eta + \lambda)(t_2 - t_1)}\right)\right]$$

$$(9.9)$$

Using the R function in Appendix 9.1, we obtain $t_2 = 79$ months. This information is useful in managing the trial. For example, if the end time or sample size required is considered too long or too large, then effort at increasing the accrual rate and decreasing withdrawals should be strategized, or the trial might be judged to be futile (Homework 9.2 through 9.4).

9.3 Modification of the Classical GS Alpha-Spending Function Procedure

The previous sections discussed monitoring the maximum information or trial duration while keeping the trial blinded. This section discusses the situation using the classical GS procedure with unblinded interim analyses of the treatment effect. As we discussed in Chapter 8, we design the classical GS procedures with a fixed maximum total information. The expected total information, however, may be reduced with chances of early termination of the trial as a result of interim analyses. The alpha-spending function approach gives us the advantage of a flexible schedule and frequency of interim analyses, with the information times calculated by the fixed maximum total information as specified in the study protocol. In the FDA's *Guidance for Industry: Adaptive Design Clinical Trials for Drugs and Biologics* (CDER and CBER 2010), they emphasized that trials with GS designs should clearly specify, in the protocol, how the alpha is to be spent during the trial. However, we also illustrated in Chapter 8 that the alpha-spending function may be altered when the observed maximum total information turns out to be different from the originally designed maximum total information. Therefore, in practice we strive to keep the actual and designed maximum total information as close as possible in order to minimize the alteration. Regardless, only when the trial continues to its final analysis without early termination will we know the actual final total information. When this occurs, the final critical value should be updated with the actual information times of all interim analyses.

When the prespecified maximum information is uncertain and a reestimation based on an interim stage data is desired, Gould and Shih (1998) suggested performing a blinded SSR before the first GS (unblinded) interim analysis, then using the reestimated maximum total information to reschedule the (classical) GS analyses.

Recently, *adaptive GS* (as opposed to classical GS) methods developed as a popular topic, in which not only the frequency and schedule of the interim analyses may change, but the maximum total information may also increase in the middle of the trial. This section and the next only discuss the case where the changes are because of administrative reasons or external information and not because of the interim data from the current trial. However, we must remain cautious that, unless there is a good reason to alter the plan designed in the protocol, the adaptive GS may not be a good idea, as illustrated in the following examples.

Example 9.2

A trial was planned with one interim analysis using an overall two-sided $\alpha = 0.05$ and the linear spending function: $\alpha(t) = \alpha t$. Thus, $\alpha(1/2) = \alpha/2 = 0.025$, which leads to $|c_1| = 2.2414$, and $\alpha(1) = \alpha = 0.05$, $|c_2| = 2.1251$. However, suppose that after $t_1 = 1/2$, the investigator, for administrative reasons, would like to add another interim analysis at $t_2 = 3/4$, with the same maximum information. We explore the available two options:

Option 1: Follow the classical GS procedure, keep the same $\alpha(t) = \alpha t$, add $t_2 = 3/4$. Then, $|c_1| = 2.2414$, $|c_2| = 2.2885$, $|c_3| = 2.2296$. All of these values can be calculated by the Lan-DeMets program and remain within the realm of the flexible alpha-spending function method. However, we emphasize that an observer will rightly make an issue of the change and ask whether the additional interim look at $t_2 = 3/4$ is "t_1-data driven." Operationally, we must justify and convince others that the additional look at $t_2 = 3/4$ resulted from an administrative reason and was not driven by the unblinded t_1-data. Along this precautionary line, keeping the DMC independent from the sponsor and keeping the sponsor blinded to the efficacy data remains vital in avoiding data-driven changes in the monitoring process.

Note that $|c_1| = 2.2414$ remains unchanged (already occurred); the new $|c_2| = 2.2885 > |c_1|$ and also > the old $|c_2|$ (2.1251). Hence, unless there is a justifiable administrative reason, adding another look at $t_2 = 3/4$ is not always logical. Furthermore, the more interim analyses we perform, the more we suffer loss of power.

Option 2: Changing to a new spending function. A skeptic would express even more suspicion if the trial switched to another spending function after the first look. For example, if we switch to spending the rest of the 0.025 type I error via the Pocock-type boundary, then the new critical values are $|c_1| = 2.2414$, $|c_2| = 2.2551$, $|c_3| = 2.2551$. (The first value is fixed because it already passed. The second and third values are the same, as characterized by the Pocock-type boundary. A program can be found in Appendix 9.2 for the above calculation.) Suppose $Z_1 = 2.22$, then the regulatory agency would also rightly feel suspicious, because the Z_1 appears so close to $|c_1| = 2.2414$. On the other hand, switching to the OBF-type boundary after t_1 would also seem foolish, because the new critical values then would be $|c_1| = 2.2414$, $|c_2| = 2.4900$, $|c_3| = 2.1564$. (Again, the first value is fixed since it already passed. The second and third values have the relationship of: $|c_2|\sqrt{3/4} = |c_3|$, as characterized by the OBF-type boundary). We also note that the boundary jumps higher at t_2.

For both options, alpha = 0.05 remains preserved. We thus conclude that changing the frequency and/or the schedule of a planned interim analysis must be performed carefully. Even without changing the fixed maximum information, using a technically correct flexible alpha-spending function method, and preserving the type I error, the boundaries can look obscured, as demonstrated in Example 9.2. Flexibility can also cause loss of efficiency, as seen with a larger critical value for the additional interim analysis.

9.4 Adaptive GS Procedure—Change Not Dependent on Unblinded Interim Data

Example 9.2 maintained no change in the maximum sample size but only added an extra interim analysis. Let us now examine a situation where we increase the maximum total information midstream of a trial. The key question for finding the boundaries to preserve the overall α is, how large is the total information increased, and how will we spend the rest of the alpha sensibly? More importantly, we need to make sure that the increase of the total information and the new schedule of the interim analyses are not driven by the unblinded interim efficacy data. We thus always ask up front, what is the purpose of the change? Although the adaptive GS procedure is flexible, change without a justifiable reason derails the spirit of the design or method flexibility. Although efficiency is not the only or most important consideration in clinical trials, we should bear in mind that design or method for flexibility can cause loss of efficiency. Again, we discuss with examples.

We first work on a one-sided test ($\alpha = 0.025$) with three planned analyses (two interim and one final analysis) based on the total information N, with boundary (c_1, c_2, c_3) given by

$$\alpha = P(Z_1 > c_1 \text{ or } Z_2 > c_2 \text{ or } Z_3 > c_3 \,|\, H_0).$$

Suppose $c_1 = z_{\alpha_1}$ with a prespecified spending function that spends the type I error rate of α_1 for the first interim analysis at t_1. After the first interim analysis, the total information N is changed to N^* ($>N$) and the new interim information at the second interim analysis is n_2^*. With this new total information, the new information times are $t_i^* = \dfrac{n_i^*}{N^*}$, for i = 1, 2, 3, as shown in Table 9.1. Note that the old schedule (t_1, t_2, 1) becomes irrelevant for calculating the new boundary.

The new critical values are obtained by

$$\alpha - \alpha_1 = P\left(Z_1 \langle Z_{\alpha_1}, Z_2 \rangle c_2 \text{ or } Z_3 > c_3 \,|\, H_0\right)$$

$$= P\left(Z_1 \langle Z_{\alpha_1}, Z_2^* \rangle c_2^* \text{ or } Z_3^* > c_3^* \,|\, H_0\right) \tag{9.10}$$

We then solve the above equation for $\left(c_2^*, c_3^*\right)$ by numerical integration of the centered multivariate normal distribution with the following covariances/correlations:

$$\text{Cov}\left(Z_1, Z_2^*\right) = \text{Corr}\left(Z_1, Z_2^*\right) = \sqrt{n_1/n_2^*} = \sqrt{t_1^*/t_2^*}$$

$$\text{Cov}\left(Z_1, Z_3^*\right) = \text{Corr}\left(Z_1, Z_3^*\right) = \sqrt{n_1/N^*} = \sqrt{t_1^*}$$

$$\text{Cov}\left(Z_2^*, Z_3^*\right) = \text{Corr}\left(Z_2^*, Z_3^*\right) = \sqrt{n_2^*/N^*} = \sqrt{t_2^*}$$

TABLE 9.1

With Two Interim Analyses and One Final
Analysis Planned Based on Total Information N

Original Schedule		Revised Schedule	
n_1	t_1	$n_1^* = n_1$	$t_1^* = \dfrac{n_1}{N^*}$
n_2	t_2	n_2^*	$t_2^* = \dfrac{n_2}{N^*}$
N	1 (Old schedule no longer relevant)	$n_3^* = N^*$	$t_3^* = 1$

Note: After the first interim analysis, the total information N is changed to N^* ($>N$).

and a specified relationship between c_2^* and c_3^*. For example, we may specify $c_2^* = c_3^*$ for the (z-value flat) Pocock-type boundary, $c_3^* = c_2^* \sqrt{\dfrac{n_2^*}{n_3^*}}$ for the (B-value flat) OBF-type boundary, or a general $c_3^* = f \times c_2^*$ for any $f \leq 1$.

Example 9.3

Consider an initial plan that defines three analyses with equal time intervals, $t_1 = 1/3$, $t_2 = 2/3$, and $t_3 = 1$. The OBF-type boundary with corresponding critical values is $(c_1 = 3.71,\ c_2 = 2.51,\ c_3 = 1.99)$. This implies that the alpha at the first interim analysis is $\alpha_1 = 0.00021$ (two-sided). Suppose that after $n_1 = 20$ patients, the sample sizes are revised to the following: $n_2 = 40$ becomes $n_2^* = 70$, $n_3 = N = 60$ becomes $n_3^* = N^* = 100$. This implies that the new schedule for analyses is $t_1^* = 0.2$, $t_2^* = 0.7$, and $t_3^* = 1$. If we continue to use the OBF-type boundary, then the revised critical values are calculated as $(c_1 = 3.71,\ c_2^* = 2.401,\ c_3^* = 2.009)$. If we switch to using the Pocock-type boundary, then the revised critical values are $(c_1 = 3.71,\ c_2^* = 2.1397,\ c_3^* = 2.1397)$.

The calculation cannot be performed using the Lan-DeMets program from Chapter 8, because their program is for the classical GS design with the alpha-spending function approach, not for the adaptive design as just described. Appendix 9.2 contains the R program used for the above calculation.

Example 9.4

Continue with the same setting of Example 9.3, but instead of modifying the schedule after the first interim analysis, we modify it after the second interim analysis: After $n_1 = 20$ and $n_2 = 40$, $n_3 = N = 60$ is revised to $n_3^* = N^* = 100$. This revision implies that the new schedule for analyses is $t_1^* = 0.2$, $t_2^* = 0.4$, and $t_3^* = 1.0$. If we continue to use the OBF-type boundary, then we calculate the revised critical values as: $(c_1 = 3.71,\ c_2^* = 2.51,\ c_3^* = 2.0289)$. Because the first two interim analyses have already occurred, the only change is their information times, not the critical values. Of course the final critical value is also altered due to the change of the correlation structure.

In summary, increasing the sample size at an interim stage changes the information fraction/time. It also changes the critical values for later analyses in order to preserve the overall type I error rate. The final critical value will most likely be larger than the original design specified in the protocol. In Examples 9.3 and 9.4 the number of analyses remained unchanged. We thus generalize the adaptation to also changing the number of analyses with the increase of the total maximum information. That is, after jth interim analysis, N changes to $N^*(>N)$, and K analyses changes to K^* analyses.

Example 9.5

Let us again look at the same scenario of having a one-sided test ($\alpha = 0.025$) with three planned analyses (two interim and one final) based on the total information N, with boundary (c_1, c_2, c_3) given by

$$\alpha = P(Z_1 > c_1 \text{ or } Z_2 > c_2 \text{ or } Z_3 > c_3 | H_0).$$

Suppose after the second interim analysis, N increases to N*, K = 3 increases to K* = 5, as shown in Table 9.2.

Similar to Equation 9.10, we obtain critical values of the new boundary by solving

$$\alpha - \alpha_1 - \alpha_2 = P\left(Z_1 \langle z_{\alpha 1}, Z_2 \langle z_{\alpha 2}, Z_3 \rangle c_3 | H_0\right)$$

$$= P\left(Z_1 \langle z_{\alpha 1}, Z_2 \langle z_{\alpha 2}, Z_3^* \rangle c_3^* \text{ or } Z_4^* \rangle c_4^* \text{ or } Z_5^* > c_5^* | H_0\right)$$

(9.11)

With the notation $Z_i^* = Z_i, n_i^* = n_i$ for $i = 1, 2$, we solve the above equation for (c_3^*, c_4^*, c_5^*) by numerical integration of the centered multivariate normal distribution with the following covariances/correlations:

$$\text{Cov}\left(Z_i^*, Z_j^*\right) = \text{Corr}\left(Z_i^*, Z_j^*\right) = \sqrt{n_i^* / n_j^*} = \sqrt{t_i^* / t_j^*} \quad i, j = 1, \ldots, 5$$

and a specified relationship among c_3^*, c_4^* and c_5^*. Similar to the previous setting, we may specify $c_5^* = c_4^* = c_3^*$ for the (z-value flat) Pocock-type boundary, $c_j^* = c_3^* \sqrt{\dfrac{n_3^*}{n_j^*}}$ ($j = 4, 5$) for the (B-value flat) OBF-type boundary, or a general constraint $c_j^* = f_j \times c_3^*$ for any $f_5 \leq f_4 \leq 1$.

TABLE 9.2

With Two Interim Analyses and One Final Analysis Planned Based on Total Information N

Original Schedule		Revised Schedule	
n_1	t_1	$n_1^* = n_1$	$t_1^* = \dfrac{n_1}{N^*}$
n_2	t_2	$n_2^* = n_2$	$t_2^* = \dfrac{n_2}{N^*}$
N	1 (old schedule no longer relevant)	n_3^*	$t_3^* = \dfrac{n_3^*}{N^*}$
		n_4^*	$t_4^* = \dfrac{n_4^*}{N^*}$
		$n_5^* = N^*$	$t_5^* = 1$

Note: After the second interim analysis, the total information N is changed to N* (>N) and total analyses K = 3 is changed to K* = 5.

Example 9.5 (Continued)

Consider again the initial plan to have three equally spaced analyses at $t_1 = 1/3$, $t_2 = 2/3$, and $t_3 = 1$. The OBF-type boundary with corresponding critical values is then $(c_1 = 3.71, c_2 = 2.51, c_3 = 1.99)$. This implies that $\alpha_1 + \alpha_2 = 0.0121$ (two-sided). Suppose that after $n_1 = 20$ and $n_2 = 40$ patients, we revise the sample sizes and frequency of analyses to the following: $n_3 = N = 60$ becomes $n_3^* = 100$, $n_4^* = 120$, and $n_5^* = N^* = 150$. This further implies the new schedule for analyses as $t_1^* = 2/15$, $t_2^* = 4/15$, $t_3^* = 10/15$, $t_4^* = 12/15$, and $t_5^* = 1$. If we continue to use the OBF-type boundary, then we calculate the revised critical values as $(c_1 = 3.71, c_2 = 2.51, c_3^* = 2.592, c_4^* = 2.366, c_5^* = 2.116)$. If we switch to using the Pocock-type boundary, then we find the revised critical values as $(c_1 = 3.71, c_2 = 2.51, c_3^* = 2.274, c_4^* = 2.274, c_5^* = 2.274)$. We further note a jump in the OBF-type boundary in the new schedule at t_3^*. We have seen this kind of jump previously (Option 2 of Example 9.2 in this chapter; Practice 8.4 in Chapter 8).

Final Note: As we noted earlier, discussion of adaptive designs, including adaptive GS procedures, in which the change of the total maximum information depends on the unblinded interim-effect size remains beyond the scope of this book. The FDA's *Guidance for Industry Adaptive Design Clinical Trials for Drugs and Biologics* (CDER and CBER 2010) specifically states that the adaptation with sample size changes based on interim-effect size estimates is a new development in clinical trial methodology and remains in the class of *adaptive designs whose properties are less understood.* If we were considering such an adaptive design, then and importantly, we would need to pay particular attention to the following issues: controlling the study-wide type I error rate, statistical bias in estimates of treatment effect associated with the study design adaptations, potential for increased type II error rate (i.e., loss of power), role of trial simulation in adaptive design planning and evaluation, and the role of a prospective statistical analysis plan.

Appendix 9.1

R function to solve for t_2 in Equation 9.9

```
# Monitoring time to study end at an interim analysis of an
      event-driven trial
# Input: n1 = number of patients at the interim analysis
      (first cohort)
#   t1 = time of the interim analysis
```

```
#   n2 = number of patients yet to enroll after the time of
        interim analysis (second cohort)
#   lambda = estimated event rate
#   nta = estimated loss-to-follow-up rate
#   d1 = number of events occurred at the interim analysis in
        the first cohort
#   d2 = number of additional events yet to occur after the
        interim analysis
#   loss = number of patients lost-to-followup before observing
        event in the first cohort
#   tr = enroll period of time from t1 for the second cohort

bisect <- function(n1 = 111,n2 = 119,lambda = 16/(65*12),nta =
    10/(65*12),t1 = 18, d1 = 16, d2 = 104,loss = 10, tr = 42,
    e = 0.001) {
 a = tr
 b = 5*tr
 for(i in 1:100){
   f = function(x) {
   lam_nta = lambda+nta
     Qa = (n1-d1-loss)*(lambda/lam_nta)*
          (1-exp(0-lam_nta*(x-t1)))
     Qb = (n2*lambda/lam_nta)*(1-(exp(0-lam_nta*(x-tr))-
          exp(0-lam_nta*(x-t1)))/(lam_nta*(tr-t1)))
     d2-Qa-Qb
     }
   if (f(a)*f(b) < 0 & abs(f(a)-f(b))>e) {
      c = (a+b)/2
      if (f(c)*f(a)<0) b = c
      else a = c
    }
    g = cbind(i,c, a, b)
  }
    g
}
# Run the example
bisect()
```

Appendix 9.2

R program for adaptive GS procedure—change does not depend on unblinded interim data

```
# Written by Yong Lin at the Biostatistics Department Rutgers
    School of Public Health
# See example runs and lecture notes for input notation
# Need to Load package mvtnorm first
```

```
Library(mvtnorm)
c.values.adapt <- function(n.new, fi.new = rep(1,length(n.
    new)), n.old, C.old, alpha = 0.05, side = 1) {
  set.seed(501)
  j <- length(n.old)
  k <- length(n.new)
  n <- c(n.old, n.new+n.old[j])
  cor.mat <- n%o% (1/n)
  cor.mat[lower.tri(cor.mat)] <- 1/cor.mat[lower.tri(cor.mat)]
  cor.mat <- sqrt(cor.mat)

if(side = =1) {
  fun <- function(ci, fv) sapply(ci, function(x) abs(1-
    pmvnorm(upper = c(C.old, x*fv),corr = cor.mat,
            algorithm = GenzBretz(abseps = 1e-12))-alpha))
  fun2 <- function(ci, fv) sapply(ci, function(x)
    1-pmvnorm(upper = c(C.old, x*fv),corr = cor.mat,
            algorithm = GenzBretz(abseps = 1e-12))-alpha)
}
else if (side = =2) {
  fun <- function(ci, fv) sapply(ci, function(x)abs(1-
    pmvnorm(lower = -c(C.old, x*fv),upper = c(C.old, x*fv),
            corr = cor.mat,algorithm = GenzBretz(abseps =
                      1e-12))-alpha))
  fun2 <- function(ci, fv) sapply(ci, function(x)1-
    pmvnorm(lower = -c(C.old, x*fv),upper = c(C.old, x*fv),
            corr = cor.mat,algorithm = GenzBretz(abseps =
                      1e-12))-alpha)
}

c.val <- optimize(f = fun,interval = c(0,10),fv = fi.new,tol =
    1e-9)$minimum
c.val2 <- uniroot(f = fun2,interval = c(0,10),fv = fi.new,tol
    = 1e-9)
Ci<- c.val*fi.new
names(C.old) <- paste('C',1:j,'.old',sep = '')
names(Ci) <- paste('C',1:k,'.new',sep = '')
ti <- n/n[j+k]

if(j = =1) alpha.left <- alpha - (1-pnorm(C.old))
else alpha.left <- alpha - (1-pmvnorm(upper = C.old, corr =
    cor.mat[1:j,1:j]))
  return(list(C = c.val,C2 = c.val2,cut_value = c(C.old,Ci),
    corr = cor.mat, information_time = ti,alpha =
    c(alpha,alpha.left)))
}
# Chapter9-Example2-option2
  # switch to Pocock type
```

```
c.values.adapt(n.new = c(30-20,40-20),fi.new = c(1,1),n.old =
    c(20), C.old = c(2.2414), side = 2)
  # switch to OBF type
c.values.adapt(n.new = c(30-20,40-20),fi.new =
    c(1,sqrt(30/40)),n.old = c(20), C.old = c(2.2414),
    side = 2)
# Chapter9-Example3
# switch to OBF type
c.values.adapt(n.new = c(70-20,100-20),fi.new =
    c(1,sqrt(70/100)),n.old = c(20),C.old = c(3.71), side = 2)
# Chapter9-Example4
c.values.adapt(n.new = c(100-40),fi.new = c(1),n.old =
    c(20,40),C.old = c(3.71,2.51), side = 2)
# Chapter9-Example5
c.values.adapt(n.new = c(100-40,120-40,150-40),fi.new =
    c(1,sqrt(100/120),sqrt(100/150)),n.old = c(20,40),C.old =
    c(3.71,2.51), side = 2)
```

Homework 9.1

Prove Equation 9.1.

Homework 9.2

Refer to Example 9.1. Vary the patient early withdrawal rate to different levels: 10/65, 9/65, 8/65, …, 1/65, and 0 (per patient-year). Comment on its effect on the solution of t_2.

Homework 9.3

In Equation 9.7, use the exponential model as before, $H(s) = \Pr(U > s) = e^{-\eta s}$, $f(s) = \lambda e^{-\lambda s}$. However, instead of the uniform entry pattern, use the (general) truncated exponential model:

$$g(\gamma, y) = \frac{\gamma e^{-\gamma y}}{1 - e^{-\gamma(t_R - t_1)}}, \quad \gamma \neq 0 \tag{9.12}$$

$$= 1/(t_R - t_1) \qquad \gamma = 0 \quad \text{(the uniform entry case)}$$

for $t_1 \le y \le t_R$.

Show that, for $\gamma \ne 0$,

Pr(subject j in Cohort Q_b will have event by time t_2, from time t_1)

$$
= \int_{t_1}^{t_R} \left[\int_0^{t_2-y} H(s)f(s)ds \right] g(y)dy
$$

$$
= \frac{\lambda}{(\eta+\lambda)} \left\{ e^{-\gamma t_1} - \frac{\gamma}{(\eta+\lambda-\gamma)\left[1-e^{-\gamma(t_R-t_1)}\right]} \left[e^{-(\eta+\lambda)(t_2-t_R)-\gamma t_R} - e^{-(\eta+\lambda)(t_2-t_1)-\gamma t_1} \right] \right\}
$$

Homework 9.4

Refer to the formula $d_2 = E_a + E_b$, where d_2 is the additional total number of events expected by time t_2; E_a and E_b are given by Equations 9.6 and 9.8, respectively. Assume the same exponential models for the primary event and loss to follow-up and uniform enrollment as in Equation 9.9. For a maximum duration trial (t_2 is fixed) to reach a certain number of events (d_1 and d_2) determined by power, write an R program (similar to the one in Appendix 9.1) to solve for the required number of subjects, n.

Homework 9.5

Use the R program c.values.adapt in Appendix 9.2 to perform the following adaptive GS design:

A trial was designed with a maximum total sample size of 120 subjects with six equally spaced analyses planned (five interim and one final) using the Pocock-type boundary: (2.453758, 2.453758, 2.453758, 2.453758, 2.453758, 2.453758) to control two-sided alpha = 0.05.

a. After the third interim analysis, the investigator wishes to change the plan and would like to conduct four additional analyses with the following revised sample sizes: 80, 100, 130, 150 (instead of the original three at 80, 100, 120), and continue to use the Pocock-type boundary. Assume the change occurred due to some administrative reason. Find and discuss the new boundary.

b. Suppose that, after the second interim analysis, the investigator wishes to change the plan and would like to conduct only two additional analyses with the sample sizes set at 80 and 100 (instead of the original four at 60, 80, 100 and 120). Continue to use the Pocock-type boundary. Assume the change occurred due to some administrative reason. Find and discuss the new boundary.

(This exercise explores how flexible the adaptive GS procedure can be by using the R program c.values.adapt. We do not suggest that anyone should conduct a study in such a fashion without a justifiable, administrative reason.)

References

CDER and CBER (US Department of Health and Human Services, Food and Drug Administration, Center for Drug Evaluation and Research and Center for Biologics Evaluation and Research). (2010). *Guidance for Industry: Adaptive Design Clinical Trials for Drugs and Biologics.* http://www.fda.gov/downloads/drugs/guidancecomplianceregulatoryinformation/guidances/ucm201790.pdf (accessed on March 30, 2014).

Gould AL and Shih WJ. (1992). Sample size reestimation without unblinding for normally distributed outcomes with unknown variance. *Communications in Statistics (A)* 21: 2833–2853.

Gould AL and Shih WJ. (1998). Modifying the design of ongoing trials without unblinding. *Statistics in Medicine* 17: 89–100.

Proschan MA, Lan KKG, and Wittes JT. (2006). *Statistical Monitoring of Clinical Trials: A Unified Approach.* New York: Springer.

Shih WJ. (1992). Sample size reestimation in clinical trials. In *Biopharmaceutical Sequential Statistical Applications*; Peace, KE (Ed.), New York: Marcel Dekker, 285–301.

10

Missing Data

10.1 Introduction

Missing data are ubiquitous in clinical trials. Consider a randomized clinical trial that compares two treatment groups with respect to a continuous outcome, y, such as blood pressure, cholesterol level, CD4 counts, pain score, forced expiratory volume in one second (FEV_1), glomerular filtration rate (GFR), hemoglobin A1c (HbA1c), or bone mineral density (BMD). Repeated measurements are often taken during the study, but the outcome at the end of the study, change from baseline, is the main interest here (as opposed to, e.g., the rate of change). A common problem in the analysis of such experiments is the data missing from subjects who drop out before the predetermined study termination, although intermittent missing values may also occur due to occasionally skipped visits. Missing data, especially when a substantial amount appears in a randomized trial, diminishes the merits of the randomization and can invalidate as well as cause loss of efficiency of the trial. (The topic of statistical efficiency was discussed in Chapter 2.) Ethically, the design of a clinical trial has to permit patients to withdraw for unfavorable reasons such as death, adverse reactions, intolerable treatment or procedure, lack of improvement, etc. However, the design and conduct of every clinical trial can and should encourage patients with favorable outcomes such as early recovery to remain in the study to achieve the full benefit of the treatment. In 2010, the National Research Council (NRC) published a report to provide recommendations regarding the design, conduct, and analysis of studies to minimize the possible dropouts and the impact of missing data due to dropouts (NRC 2010). We should first bear in mind that no single analytical method can recover the information lost in the missing data, hence we should make it a priority in trial design and conduct to limit missing data (Little et al. 2012a,b).

We should also distinguish *withdrawal from the study treatment* and *withdrawal from the study follow-up*. For ethical reasons, patients are allowed to withdraw from the study treatment at will at any time and investigators have the obligation to withdraw the study treatment when injury to the patient seems likely (see Chapter 1). However, it is important to keep the patient in the trial by providing follow-up visits and collecting key data from patients who have discontinued the study treatment. This continuing follow-up is beneficial to patients as well as for furthering the knowledge of the experimental treatment; it should be explained to all patients in their informed consent before randomization.

10.2 Question to Answer: Causal Estimand

In the beginning of Chapter 5, we pointed out that all data analysis has to be tied to the study design, even more importantly to the study objective, and subsequently also to the interpretation of the results. This statement is especially true when a clinical trial is facing the problem of missing data due to dropouts. Because the withdrawal of a patient occurs after randomization, the key feature to deriving unbiased causality of treatment effect by the randomization scheme is being compromised. We need to consider the question in a randomized trial in terms of the estimand. *Estimand* is a term used in the literature of causality. When applied to clinical trials, it is the summary quantity of the outcome measure(s) under study for the defined period of time, which addresses the inference for the target population. For example, consider a trial in which the primary outcome measure is the change in the pain score from baseline to 12 weeks after the initiation of treatment. The estimand of interest might be the difference in the mean change in the pain score at Week 12 between the target and control populations. An estimate of this parameter is the difference in sample means for participants in the treatment group and participants in the control group. This estimate is unbiased if the treatment assignment is random and there are no missing data. The goal is to attribute the difference between the treatment and the control to the causal effect of the intervention. However, with missing data present or rescue medication taken, more issues need to be considered, addressed, and resolved.

The choice of estimand involves both the endpoint as well as the population of interest. Although there are several options, we look at the three main categories of estimands that are the most commonly used for analyses in clinical trials:

1. The *intention-to-treat* (ITT) estimand, for example, the difference in mean change from baseline for all randomized participants, irrespective of taking other treatment (for tolerance alleviation or compliance): The ITT estimand is a summary of the effect of randomization to treatment. There are several aspects of this estimand that should be noted. First, all randomized subjects need to

have the outcome measure to support this estimand. For a survival study, time to death or (random) right censoring due to staggered entry is always observable, hence this estimand is usually achievable. For a trial with, for example, pain score, HbA1c, BMD, or blood pressure as the endpoint, if one can define response versus nonresponse based on a threshold of the measures, and regard all the unfavorable events that cause patients' discontinuation of the treatment as treatment failures, then either the binary "response/nonresponse" or the "time-to-treatment failure" endpoints can also support this estimand. However, the endpoint is then altered from a continuous measure. Another scenario is that the original continuous measure is desired, and the patients who discontinued the study treatment are still followed up on, with measurements collected until the end of the study. The ITT estimand is still achievable, but the original meaning of the treatment groups is altered to *treatment policy or strategy groups*, which include the concomitant therapies—for example, standard care and rescue medication—that patients receive together with, or after discontinuation of, the study treatment. This may not be a suitable interpretation or option in a regulatory setting, because it is the test treatment that is seeking regulatory approval, not the treatment policy/strategy.

The NRC (2010) report emphasizes designing trials to prevent or minimize missing data. In many situations, this involves constructing an appropriate endpoint, as the above discussion alluded to. In the example of pain studies, permitting the use of rescue medication is often a useful method to keep patients in the study. However, using a rescue medication would obscure the next pain score measured. For this reason, the FDA's guidance (CDER 2014) on pain studies states that "pain can be assessed just before the administration of rescue medication and these data carried over to the next scheduled assessment time. Alternatively, rescue medication can be limited so that none is permitted within a prespecified time before a pain assessment." The above suggestions are useful and are also applicable to other situations where rescue medication is often used. However, they also have limitations. For example, the daily pain score assessment is usually done by the patient: he or she recalls pain from the last 24 hours and scores it with a device according to a protocol-defined schedule (e.g., each morning after getting up). But rescue medication, if needed, may be taken by the patient as prescribed at any time. Another meaningful way to resolve the issue is to ask the patient to recall specifically the *worst* pain in the last 24 hours, called the *daily worst pain score* (DWPS). We then calculate the average of the DWPS each week and use the change of weekly average of DWPS from baseline as the primary endpoint.

In summary, for an ITT estimand, all patients are analyzed according to the treatment groups that they were randomized to at the beginning of the trial, regardless of off-study treatment or initiation of other treatment. This estimand essentially requires no missing data. We should consider proper ways to design a trial to prevent missing data to support this estimand. If many missing data occur, then the ITT estimand must be modified to still provide valid inference. Other possible (modified ITT, in a sense) estimands are discussed in the following.

2. The *as control treatment* (ACT) estimand, for example, the difference in mean change from baseline at the end of the study, assuming all the treatment group dropouts evolve as the control completers for the remaining study duration. Little and Yao (1998) considered a case where the control may be given a placebo. Multiple imputations can be carried out by repeatedly sampling outcomes from the predictive model constructed by the control/placebo group to replace the missing data for all dropouts. This (multiple) imputation can shed light on what could be the outcome value for individuals who stopped the study medication.

3. The *as assigned treatment* (AAT) estimand, for example, the difference in mean change from baseline at the end of the study, assuming all the treatment dropouts remained on their assigned study treatment evolution (with or without modification) for the remaining study duration. The need for possible modification for discontinuations due to AEs or lack of efficacy is discussed in Section 10.7. Multiple imputations can be carried out by repeatedly sampling outcomes from the predictive model to replace the missing data in the corresponding treatment group. Most of the literature on methods for dealing with missing data is in this category. The imputation for the AAT estimand is discussed in detail in Sections 10.5 through 10.7.

10.3 Missing Data Patterns and Mechanisms

For the ACT and AAT estimands, where imputation of missing data is required, we need to understand the process that causes the missing data. Let us first contrast the situations of complete data and incomplete data. Let $Y = \{y_{ij}\}$ denote the complete-data matrix of the measurement, possibly observed incompletely. We can write it as $Y = (Y_{obs}, Y_{mis})$, where Y_{obs} is the observed part and Y_{mis} is the missing part. Furthermore, let $M = \{m_{ij}\}$ denote the missing-data indicator matrix that identifies whether y_{ij} is observed or missing. M is usually called the *missing data pattern* (Rubin 1976). The key to the analysis of missing data is to be aware that M is part of the random variables that need to be considered, in addition to Y when missing data is present. The observed "data set" is $V = (Y_{obs}, M)$, not Y_{obs} alone. This is similar to the censoring indicator variable for the survival data analysis. (In fact, missing data and censored data both belong to the larger class of incomplete data.) In addition, the underlying reason for the missing data or dropouts is also an important part of the information that should be considered in the analysis. For some approaches, as we shall see later, M incorporates the cause and/or time of the missing data.

For simplicity, we use the bracket [Y; θ] to denote the distribution of a random variable Y with parameter θ. Because the missing data pattern M is a part of the data, we need to consider the joint distribution of Y and M, [Y, M]. We may add in other predefined baseline covariates X, such as treatment group ID. Because the focus here is on missing outcomes, X is assumed to be always observed. When X is the treatment group, the parameter θ in [Y|X; θ] is the treatment effect, which is the parameter of primary interest. In the following, X is omitted for simplicity, but all results are still applicable when X is conditioned on.

The joint distribution [Y, M] can be factored into the conditional and marginal distributions as

$$[Y, M] = [M|Y; \varphi]\,[Y; \theta] \qquad (10.1)$$

or

$$[Y, M] = [Y|M; \theta_M]\,[M] \qquad (10.2)$$

Analysis methods with the first type of factorization are said to use the *selection model approach* and analysis methods with the second type of factorization are said to use *pattern-mixture model* (PMM) *approach* (Little 1995). In the first factorization, the conditional distribution [M|Y; φ] with parameter φ characterizes how the missing data depends on the outcome measure Y and is called the *missing data process* or *missing data mechanism* (MDM). In the second factorization, the conditional distribution [Y|M; θ_M] is the conditional distribution given the missing data pattern, with parameter θ_M. Note that we write explicitly the associated parameters for clear inference and interpretation in each approach. With the selection model approach one has to specify an explicit model for the MDM [M|Y; φ] to make an appropriate inference for θ. It is a useful research tool for performing simulation studies with missing data, but it is difficult to apply to a real data analysis because [M|Y; φ] may involve the missing data Y_m. The example in the next section gives a simple illustration for θ and φ. Shih (1992) and Diggle and Shih (1993) contain a more advanced example of $[Y; \theta]$ and $[M|Y; \varphi]$ (Homework 10.1a and 10.1c). The pattern-mixture model approach, on the other hand, has no such concern in $[M]$. However, the parameter of $[Y|M; \theta_M]$ is conditioning on the missing data pattern. We need to combine θ_M over the patterns M to obtain the parameter θ of the marginal $[Y]$; see Equation 10.13 for an illustration.

10.4 Ignorability and Nonignorability of Missing Data

All the ITT, ACT, and AAT estimands make inferences about θ. The inference should be based on the entire observed data $V = (Y_{obs}, M)$, not on Y_{obs} alone. However, because it is generally simpler and easier to ignore M and to make the inference based on Y_{obs} alone, a fundamental question is, when is it appropriate to ignore M and base the analysis on Y_{obs} alone? The first type of factorization (Equation 10.1) is useful in answering the above question: whether the missing data is ignorable or not. Actually, to be precise we should say, whether or not the mechanism of the process or mechanism producing the missing data is ignorable in making the inference regarding the parameter θ of the hypothetical complete data distribution.

The exact answer to this question involves the definitions of *missing completely at random* (MCAR), *missing at random* (MAR), and *distinct parameters* given by Rubin (1976). Details are given in Appendices 10.1 and 10.2 of this chapter. In brief:

> If the MDM is not related to the observed or potential outcome of the patient, then MCAR may be assumed. Using the notation in Equation 10.1, $[M|Y] = [M]$. Examples include patients moving away, the study ending, and late enrollment of patients being administratively "censored." When MCAR is applicable, the inference based on Y_0 alone is appropriate. The usual two-sample t-test based on the sample means and the method of *generalized estimating equations* (GEE) for unbalanced clustered data including repeated measures (Liang and Zeger 1986) requires the assumption of MCAR because these methods are based on sampling distributions.
>
> MAR may be assumed if the patient's withdrawal from the study is solely due to the observed outcome but not the current unobserved or future potential outcomes. Using the notation in Equation 10.1, $[M|Y] = [M|Y_{obs}]$. When MAR is applicable, the likelihood-based inference based on Y_0 alone is appropriate, provided that the parameter of interest, θ, and the missing data process parameter, φ, are distinct. The method of *weighted estimation equations* (Robins, Rotnitzky, and Zhao 1995; Paik 1997), the mixed-effect models (Laird and Ware 1982) in SAS PROC

MIXED, and the multiple imputation method (Rubin 1998) in SAS PROC MI (Yuan 2001) all require the MAR assumption.

Not missing at random (NMAR), or missing not at random (MNAR), is when the patient's withdrawal from the study is dependent on the current unobserved or future potential outcomes. Using the notation of Equation 10.1, $[M|Y] = [M|Y_o, Y_m]$ with particular reference to Y_m. More discussion is given in Appendix 10.5. Now, we provide a simple example from Choi and Lu (1995) to illustrate the concept of NMAR and show how bias can occur under NMAR if the MDM is ignored.

Example 10.1

Consider the case of comparing two randomized treatment groups, X and Y, with respect to a binary endpoint, with 1 being response and 0 being nonresponse. Let the response rate of treatment group X be p_x and that of treatment group Y be p_y. In notation, $p_x = E(X) = Pr(X = 1)$; the same is true for p_y. We are interested in $\theta = p_x - p_y$. Suppose that there is a mechanism that will cause the outcome to go missing, depending on whether the outcome is a response or a nonresponse. The MDM is indexed by the parameters (φ_0, φ_1), where $\varphi_0 = Pr(\text{missing } X|X = 0) = Pr(\text{missing } Y|Y = 0)$, and $\varphi_1 = Pr(\text{missing } X|X = 1) = Pr(\text{missing } Y|Y = 1)$. Note that, for simplicity, the MDM is assumed to be the same for both treatment groups. In this setting, $|\varphi_0 - \varphi_1|$ is an indication of the degree of NMAR, compared to MAR/MCAR, where $\varphi_0 = \varphi_1$. We now examine what the bias would be if the MDM were ignored by using the difference of the sample proportions, $\hat{P}_x - \hat{P}_y$.

Suppose X_i, $i = 1, ..., n_x$, and Y_j, $j = 1, ..., n_y$ are observed. (n_x and n_y are also random variables.) Note that $Pr(X \text{ is observed}) = 1 - Pr(X \text{ is missing})$

$$= 1 - [Pr(X \text{ is missing}|X = 0)P(X = 0) + Pr(X \text{ is missing}|X = 1)P(X = 1)]$$

$$= 1 - [\varphi_0(1 - p_x) + \varphi_1 p_x]$$

$$\equiv \pi_x$$

Likewise, $Pr(Y \text{ is observed}) = 1 - [\varphi_0(1 - p_y) + \varphi_1 p_y] \equiv \pi_y$.
The expected value of $\hat{P}_x$ is obtained as follows

$$E(\hat{P}_x) = E\left(n_x^{-1}\sum_{i=1}^{n_x} X_i\right)$$

$$= E\left\{E\left(n_x^{-1}\sum_{i=1}^{n_x} X_i \mid n_x\right)\right\}$$

$$= E\left\{n_x^{-1}\, E\left(\sum_{i=1}^{n_x} X_i \mid n_x\right)\right\}$$

$$= E\left\{n_x^{-1}\sum_{i=1}^{n_x} E(X_i \mid n_x)\right\} \qquad (10.3)$$

In Equation 10.3, $E(X_i \mid n_x) = \Pr(X_i = 1 \mid X_i \text{ is observed})$

$$= \frac{\Pr\left(X_i \text{ is observed} \mid X_i = 1\right)\Pr\left(X_i = 1\right)}{\Pr\left(X_i \text{ is observed}\right)}$$

$$= \frac{(1-\varphi_1)p_x}{\pi_x}$$

Plug this into Equation 10.3 to obtain $E(\hat{p}_x) = \dfrac{(1-\varphi_1)p_x}{\pi_x}$. Likewise, $E(\hat{p}_y) = \dfrac{(1-\varphi_1)p_y}{\pi_y}$.

Hence, $E(\hat{p}_x - \hat{p}_y) = \dfrac{(1-\varphi_1)p_x}{\pi_x} - \dfrac{(1-\varphi_1)p_y}{\pi_y}$

$$= \frac{\pi_y(1-\varphi_1)p_x - \pi_x(1-\varphi_1)p_y}{\pi_x \pi_y} \qquad (10.4)$$

$$= \frac{(1-\varphi_0)(1-\varphi_1)(p_x - p_y)}{\pi_x \pi_y}$$

Equation 10.4 shows a bias multiplier factor $= \dfrac{(1-\varphi_0)(1-\varphi_1)}{\pi_x \pi_y} \cdot \hat{p}_x - \hat{p}_y$ is an unbiased estimator of $\theta = p_x - p_y$ if $\varphi_0 = \varphi_1$ (MCAR, the multiplier factor equals 1), or if $\theta = 0$ (no treatment effect).

In practice, the validity of the assumption of MCAR or MAR requires careful examination of the missing data information and a strong belief in the reasons given for patients' withdrawal. Because the inference depends on the missing data model, which is not a verifiable object from the observed data, a prudent strategy is to do a *sensitivity analysis*, as suggested in the ICH-E9 guideline (EMEA 1998). That is, we should specify a set of plausible models of the MDM in the protocol and investigate the sensitivity of the results of the analysis to the different models and methods of handling missing values. In the following, we discuss the multiple imputation method under the MAR assumption (Sections 10.5 and 10.6) and that under a particular NMAR model assumption (Section 10.7).

10.5 Analysis under the MAR Assumption by Multiple Imputation

The method of multiple imputation (MI) is perhaps the most commonly used technique to address the AAT estimand when the MAR assumption is attainable, as well as for the ACT estimand, which always assumes NMAR. MI can also be used for NMAR when any particular NMAR model can be explicitly expressed (see Section 10.7). The MI method in general is carried out in three steps: (a) Select a multivariate model and sample from this model to impute (fill in) the missing values G times to obtain G complete data sets; (b) For each of the G complete data sets, perform the proper analysis for complete data (such as the mixed-effects model for repeated measures or MMRM), obtaining the mean and within-imputation and between-imputation variances of the summary outcome measure; and (c) Combine the G means by incorporating the within and between-imputation variances. For example, let $\hat{\theta}_j$ be the estimate of the treatment effect θ and v_j be the estimate of the variance of $\hat{\theta}_j$ from the jth imputation. Then, the combined estimate is $\bar{\theta} = \sum_{j=1}^{G} \hat{\theta}_j/G$, and the (total) variance is

$$\sum_{j=1}^{G} v_j/G + \left(1 + G^{-1}\right)B$$

where the first term is the average within-imputation variance, $B = \dfrac{1}{G-1}\sum_{j=1}^{G}\left(\hat{\theta}_j - \bar{\theta}\right)^2$ is the between-imputation variance, and the multiplier $(1 + G^{-1})$ is a finite number correction.

For analyses with the MAR assumption, steps (a) and (c) are directly implemented in SAS PROC MI and PROC MIANALYZE. Details can be found in the SAS documentation. For analyses with a particular NMAR assumption, the imputation step (a) in SAS needs to be augmented by a specific NMAR model (Section 10.7).

The assumption of MAR may be a concern in practice. However, according to Schafer (1997) and Rubin (1998), the plausibility of the MAR assumption will be enhanced when there are sufficient covariates in the imputation model of step (a). The model in step (a) is called the "imputer's model," which can have a larger set of covariates than the complete-data analysis model in step (b) after the missing values have been imputed. The subset of covariates used for the complete-data analysis is called the "analyst's model."

10.6 Analysis of Longitudinal Data with Monotone Pattern Missing Values under MAR

For longitudinal data with missing data caused by dropouts, as is commonly the case in clinical trials, a monotone pattern is formed naturally. Specifically, consider a study with T scheduled post baseline visits. Let Y_k denote the outcome at visit k, k = 0, 1, 2, ..., T, where k = 0 is the baseline visit. Under the monotone missing data pattern, if the subject's outcome Y_k is missing at visit k, then the outcomes Y_j at the future visits j > k are also missing. For this discrete time model, let L be the follow-up time, that is, the last visit that a subject has a measurement observed. The monotone missing data pattern is then characterized by L = 0, 1, ..., T, where L = T is when the subject completes the study visits. The baseline values are assumed to always be observed. A feasible analysis in this situation is based on the factorization in Equation 10.2, that is, the PMM approach. We discuss the approach with the case where T = 4, as illustrated in Table 10.1.

With the pattern-mixture approach, the MAR condition $[M|Y] = [M|Y_{obs}]$ is equivalent to $[Y_{mis}|Y_{obs}, M] = [Y_{mis}|Y_{obs}]$. That is, the conditional distributions of the variables with missing data given observed variables are the same across the missing data pattern (see Appendix 10.4 for proof of the equivalence). For example, Table 10.1 illustrates the imputation using the pattern-mixture MAR condition $[Y_{mis}|Y_{obs}, M] = [Y_{mis}|Y_{obs}]$.

TABLE 10.1

Monotone Missing Data for T = 4 and Missing at Random Conditions with PMM

| | Y_k | | | | |
	k = 0	k = 1	k = 2	k = 3	k = 4
L = 0	x	? = $[Y_1\|Y_0,$ $L > 0]$	? = $[Y_2\|Y_0,$ $Y_1, L > 1]$	? = $[Y_3\|Y_0, Y_1,$ $Y_2, L > 2]$	? = $[Y_4\|Y_0, Y_1,$ $Y_3, L > 3]$
L = 1	x	$[Y_1\|Y_0, L = 1]$	? = $[Y_2\|Y_0,$ $Y_1, L > 1]$	? = $[Y_3\|Y_0, Y_1,$ $Y_2, L > 2]$	? = $[Y_4\|Y_0, Y_1,$ $Y_3, L > 3]$
L = 2	x	$[Y_1\|Y_0, L = 2]$	$[Y_2\|Y_0, Y_1,$ $L = 2]$	? = $[Y_3\|Y_0, Y_1,$ $Y_2, L > 2]$	? = $[Y_4\|Y_0, Y_1,$ $Y_3, L > 3]$
L = 3	x	$[Y_1\|Y_0, L = 3]$	$[Y_2\|Y_0, Y_1,$ $L = 3]$	$[Y_3\|Y_0, Y_1, Y_2,$ $L = 3]$	? = $[Y_4\|Y_0, Y_1,$ $Y_3, L > 3]$
L = 4	x	$[Y_1\|Y_0, L = 4]$	$[Y_2\|Y_0, Y_1,$ $L = 4]$	$[Y_3\|Y_0, Y_1, Y_2,$ $L = 4]$	$[Y_4\|Y_0, Y_1, Y_3,$ $L = 4]$

Note: k = study visit; L = last study visit with observed measure, describing the missing data pattern. Each row may represent one or more subjects. X denotes observed data, ? denotes missing data and is identified by the specified distribution.

Let us see how the $[Y_{mis}|Y_{obs}, M] = [Y_{mis}|Y_{obs}]$ condition identifies all the joint distributions for each pattern. For the observations with the pattern $L = 0$, only Y_0 (baseline) is observed and all other follow-up values Y_1 to Y_4 need to be imputed. Using the MAR with pattern-mixture approach

$$[Y_1, Y_2, Y_3, Y_4|Y_0, L = 0]$$

$$= [Y_1, Y_2, Y_3, Y_4|Y_0]$$

$$= [Y_4|Y_0, Y_1, Y_2, Y_3][Y_1, Y_2, Y_3|Y_0] \tag{10.5}$$

$$= [Y_4|Y_0, Y_1, Y_2, Y_3, L = 4][Y_3|Y_0, Y_1, Y_2][Y_1, Y_2|Y_0]$$

$$= [Y_4|Y_0, Y_1, Y_2, Y_3, L = 4][Y_3|Y_0, Y_1, Y_2, L \geq 3][Y_2|Y_0, Y_1][Y_1|Y_0]$$

$$= [Y_4|Y_0, Y_1, Y_2, Y_3, L = 4][Y_3|Y_0, Y_1, Y_2, L \geq 3][Y_2|Y_0, Y_1, L \geq 2][Y_1|Y_0, L \geq 1]$$

Hence, the joint distribution of $[Y_1, Y_2, Y_3, Y_4|Y_0, L = 0]$ can be estimated because all the factors on the right-hand side of Equation 10.5 can be identified from the observed data. The same factorization and application of the MAR to the variables with missing values are performed for patterns $L = 1$, 2, 3. (There are no missing data in $L = 4$.) Missing values are sampled from the predictive/conditional distributions. This is the basis for the MI method. The derivations of Equation 10.5 suggest that the imputation can be done sequentially from $[Y_1|Y_0] = [Y_1|Y_0, L \geq 1]$ to $[Y_4|Y_0, Y_1, Y_2, Y_3] = [Y_4|Y_0, Y_1, Y_2, Y_3, L = 4]$, conditioning on the previous responses as follows:

$$[Y_1|Y_0, L = 0] = [Y_1|Y_0, L > 0]$$

$$[Y_2|Y_0, Y_1, L = 1] = [Y_2|Y_0, Y_1, L > 1] \tag{10.6}$$

$$[Y_3|Y_0, Y_1, Y_2, L = 2] = [Y_3|Y_0, Y_1, Y_2, L > 2]$$

$$[Y_4|Y_0, Y_1, Y_2, Y_3, L = 3] = [Y_4|Y_0, Y_1, Y_2, Y_3, L > 3]$$

In the above, for the pattern $L = j$, the predictive/conditional distribution at the right-hand side can be obtained from the observed data in the pattern $L > j$. Missing values Y_{j+1} in the pattern $L = j$ (left-hand side) are sampled from the predictive/conditional distribution of the right-hand side, as performed by the MI procedures in SAS. In PROC MI, the sequential imputations can actually be carried out in one command (Homework 10.1b and 10.1c).

In a situation where the data has some cases with intermittent missing values, SAS PROC MI has an option to first create a monotone pattern from the intermittent missing values using the Markov chain Monte Carlo (MCMC) method before proceeding with the analysis with a monotone pattern.

The following are SAS codes to carry out MI under MAR. Assume we have a data set called "datain," which has an arbitrary missing data pattern. The covariates are age, sex, race, and treatment group (trt). Age is continuous and other covariates are categorical variables. First, we generate the monotone missing pattern:

```
proc mi data = datain out = outmono nimpute = 2 seed = 1234;
mcmc impute = monotone;
var age sex race1 race2 race3 trt Y0 Y1 Y2 Y3 Y4;
run;
```

Note that we created a design matrix (with dummy variables) for race in the above procedure (without showing the previous step of creation race1 to race3) because the MCMC procedure that is used to fill in intermittent missing values assumes multivariate normality in SAS; therefore, it cannot take categorical variables directly by the CLASS statement when mcmc is used. This step outputs the monotone pattern data "outmono." There are two copies made for "outmono" through the option "nimute = 2."

Next, perform MI on each of the copies of the "outmono" data set using the regression (conditional expectation) method.

```
proc mi data = outmono out = miout nimpute = 5 seed = 1234;
monotone method = REG;
var age sex race1 race2 race3 trt y0 y1 y2 y3 y4 y5;
run;
```

The imputation by regression is carried out sequentially in the order specified in the *Var* statement above. The conditional expectation starts from the first variable that has missing data and fills in the missing data with regression, which conditions on all the proceeding variables as factors. It is not necessary to separate the sequential imputation with multiple steps. However, when we need to augment the conditional expectation (from MAR) with additional restrictions, as in NMAR, some strategy may require separation of the sequential steps.

10.7 Analysis under a Particular NMAR Model Assumption by MI

When the assumption of MCAR or MAR cannot be made, one cannot simply "ignore M." Hence, the likelihood-based analysis based on the factorization in Equation 10.1, that is, the selection model approach, requires modeling the MDM $[M|Y_{obs}, Y_{mis}; \varphi]$. Because there are infinitely many such models and none can be verified from the observed data, no general computing program is available and a prudent strategy is to perform "sensitivity analyses" with various models. A useful subclass of NMAR, called *nonfuture dependence* (NFD) *missingness* introduced by Kenward, Molenberghs, and Thijs (2003) is given in Appendix 10.5. We discuss the specific analysis under NFD missingness in this section (Homework 10.2a).

The NFD can be formulated so that MAR is a special case of NFD. We continue the pattern-mixture approach to the analysis of data with a monotone pattern in order to make a connection between the NFD missingness and the MAR model. Continuing with the example described in Table 10.1 with T = 4, for MAR, we illustrate in Table 10.2 the NFD missingness conditions given in Appendix 10.5, Equation 10A.11.

Contrasting Tables 10.1 (MAR) and 10.2, we see that the NFD-NMAR (Table 10.2 and Equation 10A.11) is not a comprehensive set of conditions. That is, there are missing data distributions left unidentified (denoted by a double question mark in Table 10.2). In order to further identify those missing data denoted as double question marks (??) in Table 10.2, we need a further assumption that can link to Equation 10.6 under MAR as follows.

A simple way to describe the departure from MAR is by a model with a shift in the conditional means of Equation 10.6. This *mean shift model* assumption cannot be verified from the data itself. The justification for this choice is based mainly on interpretability: place a penalty on the imputed value for missing data due to unfavorable reasons such as lack of efficacy or AE. It works as follows. First, assume linear regression (i.e., conditional mean)

TABLE 10.2

Monotone Missing Data for T = 4 and Nonfuture Dependence Not Missing at Random Conditions with PMM

	Y_k				
	k = 0	k = 1	k = 2	k = 3	k = 4
L = 0	x	??	? = $[Y_2 \mid Y_0, Y_1, L \geq 1]$	? = $[Y_3 \mid Y_0, Y_1, Y_2, L \geq 2]$	? = $[Y_4 \mid Y_0, Y_1, Y_3, L \geq 3]$
L = 1	x	$[Y_1 \mid Y_0, L = 1]$	??	? = $[Y_3 \mid Y_0, Y_1, Y_2, L \geq 2]$	? = $[Y_4 \mid Y_0, Y_1, Y_3, L \geq 3]$
L = 2	x	$[Y_1 \mid Y_0, L = 2]$	$[Y_2 \mid Y_0, Y_1, L = 2]$	??	? = $[Y_4 \mid Y_0, Y_1, Y_3, L \geq 3]$
L = 3	x	$[Y_1 \mid Y_0, L = 3]$	$[Y_2 \mid Y_0, Y_1, L = 3]$	$[Y_3 \mid Y_0, Y_1, Y_2, L = 3]$	??
L = 4	x	$[Y_1 \mid Y_0, L = 4]$	$[Y_2 \mid Y_0, Y_1, L = 4]$	$[Y_3 \mid Y_0, Y_1, Y_2, L = 4]$	$[Y_4 \mid Y_0, Y_1, Y_3, L = 4]$

Note: k = study visit; L = last study visit with observed measure, describing the missing data pattern; each row may represent one or more subjects. x denotes observed data, ? denotes missing data and is identified by the specified distribution, ?? denotes the missing data and unidentified distributions (which implies that we need more assumptions, and will relate to sensitivity analysis).

models for the observed (right-hand side of Equation 10.6), which can and should be checked with the observed data:

$$E(Y_1|Y_0, L > 0) = \alpha_1 + \beta_1 Y_0$$

$$E(Y_2|Y_0, Y_1, L > 1) = \alpha_2 + \beta_{20} Y_0 + \beta_{21} Y_1 \tag{10.7}$$

$$E(Y_3|Y_0, Y_1, Y_2, L > 2) = \alpha_3 + \beta_{30} Y_0 + \beta_{31} Y_1 + \beta_{32} Y_2$$

$$E(Y_4|Y_0, Y_1, Y_2, Y_3, L > 3) = \alpha_4 + \beta_{40} Y_0 + \beta_{41} Y_1 + \beta_{42} Y_2 + \beta_{43} Y_3$$

All the intercept and slope coefficients can be estimated from the observed data. Next, to embed the MAR specification in this larger class of NMAR models, the NMAR class will be indexed by shifts in linking the dropouts with the observed conditional means. Third, assume that the shift is in the intercept, not in the slopes or the residual variances (Daniels and Hogan 2007, 240; NRC 2010, 100). That is,

$$E(Y_1|Y_0, L = 0) = (\alpha_1 + \Delta_1) + \beta_1 Y_0$$

$$= E(Y_1|Y_0, L > 0) + \Delta_1 \text{ for all } Y_0$$

$$E(Y_2|Y_0, Y_1, L = j) = (\alpha_2 + \Delta_{2j}) + \beta_{20} Y_0 + \beta_{21} Y_1$$

$$= E(Y_2|Y_0, Y_1, L > 1) + \Delta_{2j} \text{ for } j = 0, 1 \text{ and all } Y_0, Y_1$$

$$E(Y_3|Y_0, Y_1, Y_2, L = j) = (\alpha_3 + \Delta_{3j}) + \beta_{30} Y_0 + \beta_{31} Y_1 + \beta_{32} Y_2 \tag{10.8}$$

$$= E(Y_3|Y_0, Y_1, Y_2, L > 2) + \Delta_{3j} \text{ for } j = 0, 1, 2$$
$$\text{and all } Y_0, Y_1, Y_2$$

$$E(Y_4|Y_0, Y_1, Y_2, Y_3, L = j) = (\alpha_4 + \Delta_{4j}) + \beta_{40} Y_0 + \beta_{41} Y_1 + \beta_{42} Y_2 + \beta_{43} Y_3$$

$$= E(Y_4|Y_0, Y_1, Y_2, Y_3, L > 3) + \Delta_{4j} \text{ for } j = 0, 1, 2, 3$$
$$\text{and all } Y_0, Y_1, Y_2, Y_3$$

Furthermore, an additional simplification is that $\Delta_{2j} = \Delta_2$ for $j = 0, 1$; $\Delta_{3j} = \Delta_3$ for $j = 0, 1, 2$; and $\Delta_{4j} = \Delta_4$ for $j = 0, 1, 2, 3$. That is, the shift is the same across patterns for each visit with missing data. This is derived from the characteristic of the NFD missingness (Kenward, Molenberghs, and Thijs 2003); see Appendix 10.5 for more detail.

Because the regression parameters can all be estimated, the left-hand side of Equation 10.8 can also be estimated when the shift parameters $\Delta = (\Delta_1, \Delta_2, \Delta_3, \Delta_4)$ are specified. The missing data in pattern $L = j$ will be filled in sequentially with the conditional mean in Equation 10.8. Computationally, because Equation 10.8 (for NFD missing) is only a shift of Equation 10.7 (for MAR), we can utilize the MI procedure based on MAR and apply shifts to the imputed values obtained from PROC MI. Note that the shift parameters $\Delta = (\Delta_1, \Delta_2, \Delta_3, \Delta_4)$ are applied together after the process of filling in the missing data under MAR is completed through MIs. They are not involved in the process of MI with MAR. It is a nonrecursive procedure. A recursive procedure is presented by Ratitch, O'Kelly, and Tosielloc (2013), which applies the shift parameters sequentially from time point to time point while conducting the imputation. That is, perform MI for the first time point with missing data under MAR, then apply Δ_1 to the imputed values in each of the imputations. Treating these Δ_1-adjusted values as observed, perform imputation for the second time point with missing data under MAR, then apply Δ_2 to the imputed values of the second time point. Treating these Δ_2-adjusted values as observed, perform imputation for the third time point with missing data under MAR, etc. Note that, to avoid compounding MIs when there are many time points with missing data, sometimes it is necessary to limit imputations to only the first time point, then for each of these imputations a single imputation is performed for all subsequent time points. This is called single adjustment algorithm. Peng (2015) examines these algorithms (nonsequential, sequential, and single adjustment) and concludes that nonsequential and single adjustment work better than the sequential algorithm. A homework exercise is to compare these three procedures (Homework 10.2b).

Analytically, we can show how to obtain the marginal means of the outcome at each visit in each pattern and the marginal mean at the final visit over the patterns. Denote $\mu_k^{(j)} = E(Y_k \mid L = j)$. It follows from Equation 10.8 that for each follow-up visit post baseline, we can sequentially obtain the pattern-specific marginal means:

$$\mu_1^{(0)} = E(Y_1 \mid L = 0) = (\alpha_1 + \Delta_1) + \beta_1 \mu_0^{(0)} \tag{10.9}$$

where $\mu_0^{(0)} = E(Y_1 \mid L = 0)$ is estimated directly from the pattern-specific observed data.

$$\mu_2^{(j)} = E(Y_2 \mid L = j) = (\alpha_2 + \Delta_2) + \beta_{20} \mu_0^{(j)} + \beta_{21} \mu_1^{(j)} \text{ for } j = 0, 1 \tag{10.10}$$

where $\mu_0^{(0)}, \mu_0^{(1)}, \mu_1^{(1)}$ are estimated directly from the observed data, and $\mu_1^{(0)}$ is obtained from Equation 10.9.

$$\mu_3^{(j)} = E(Y_3 \mid L = j) = (\alpha_3 + \Delta_3) + \beta_{30} \mu_0^{(j)} + \beta_{31} \mu_1^{(j)} + \beta_{32} \mu_2^{(j)} \text{ for } j = 0, 1, 2 \tag{10.11}$$

where $\mu_0^{(0)}, \mu_0^{(1)}, \mu_0^{(2)}, \mu_1^{(1)}, \mu_1^{(2)}, \mu_2^{(2)}$ are estimated directly from the observed data, $\mu_1^{(0)}$ is obtained from Equation 10.9, and $\mu_2^{(0)}, \mu_2^{(1)}$ are obtained from Equation 10.10.

$$\mu_4^{(j)} = E(Y_4 \mid L = j) = (\alpha_4 + \Delta_4) + \beta_{40} \mu_0^{(j)} + \beta_{41} \mu_1^{(j)} + \beta_{42} \mu_2^{(j)} + \beta_{43} \mu_3^{(j)} \text{ for } j = 0, 1, 2, 3 \tag{10.12}$$

where $\mu_0^{(0)}, \mu_0^{(1)}, \mu_0^{(2)}, \mu_0^{(3)}, \mu_1^{(1)}, \mu_1^{(2)}, \mu_1^{(3)}, \mu_2^{(2)}, \mu_2^{(3)}, \mu_3^{(3)}$ are estimated directly from the observed data, while $\mu_1^{(0)}$ is obtained from Equation 10.9, $\mu_2^{(0)}, \mu_2^{(1)}$ are obtained from Equation 10.10, and $\mu_3^{(0)}, \mu_3^{(1)}, \mu_3^{(2)}$ are obtained from Equation 10.11. Using the notation of Equation 10.2, $\theta_M = \left\{\mu_4^{(j)}, j = 0, 1, 2, 3\right\}$.

In many clinical trials, the primary interest is on the marginal mean of the final visit at the last time point T. For the illustration of T = 4,

$$\theta = E(Y_4) = \sum_{j=0}^{4} \omega_j E(Y_4 \mid L = j) = \sum_{j=0}^{4} \omega_j \mu_4^{(j)} \qquad (10.13)$$

where $\omega_j = P(L = j)$ is estimated by the proportion of subjects in the pattern $L = j$.

The shift parameters $\Delta = (\Delta_1, \Delta_2, \Delta_3, \Delta_4)$ can be varied over a space of Δ, $D(\Delta)$, to perform sensitivity analysis to see how the result changes from the MAR case where $\Delta = (0, 0, 0, 0)$. The scale of departure from MAR can be determined in different ways. One metric is to use the residual standard deviation of Y_k given $(Y_0, \dots, Y_{k-1})$, RSD_k, which can be obtained from the imputed complete data under MAR before engaging the NMAR model. For example, we may set the maximum range of departure from MAR at visit k equal to a factor f_k of RSD_k. If prior belief about the value of Δ_k is confined to being within $f_k \times RSD_k$, then $D(\Delta) = (f_1 \times RSD_1, \dots, f_4 \times RSD_4)$. Each missing value at visit k is then replaced with $E(Y_k \mid Y_0, \dots, Y_{k-1}, L > k-1) + Unif \times f_k \times RSD_k$, where $E(Y_k \mid Y_0, \dots, Y_{k-1}, L > k-1)$ is estimated from the imputation steps under MAR and Unif is a random value from the uniform (0, 1) distribution. For example, Daniels and Hogan (2007) used $f_k = 1$ for all k = 1, …, T. It is conceivable that $RSD_k \geq RSD_{k'}$ for k < k′, because fewer Ys are included in the regression model at earlier time points. This also indicates that greater penalties are more likely to be placed on the earlier dropouts than later ones, which is reasonable. Another metric is to use the STD_k (pooled standard deviation at time point k). STD_k would be increasing over time, contrary to RSD_k. It is also reasonable to add more "penalty" to missing data because the treatment effect would be wearing off more and more as time goes on after withdrawal. Peng (2015) also examines the sensitivity analysis using the two different metrics and recommends RSD over STD (Homework 10.2b).

For simplicity, Tables 10.1 and 10.2 and all illustrations above are performed without regard to the treatment group. In practice we would include the treatment group as a covariate in the regression model instead of performing the MI separately for each treatment group. When the missing values are multiply imputed by the NMAR model, other restrictions may also be considered. For example, for a pain score that ranges from 0 to 10, the imputed value should also be restricted in this range. Suppose that a clinical interpretation of withdrawal due to ineffective therapy means that the missing value should not be better than the baseline value; the imputed value should then also adopt this restriction.

10.8 Use Reason for Withdrawal and Follow-Up Time to Form the Missing Data Pattern and Sensitivity Analyses

The above illustration uses T = 4, thus the monotone pattern is L = 0, 1, ..., 4, which can easily be generalized. The pattern can also be set up to incorporate other factors than just using the discrete follow-up time L, the last visit with observation before withdrawal. For example, it is very reasonable to use the reason of withdrawal as one factor in addition to L. In this case, we can use the same *shifting factor* f_k across visits, but vary them for different reasons for withdrawal. It is conceivable that for analyzing the efficacy outcome, we apply a larger shifting factor value for the withdrawal due to lack of efficacy ($f_1 = f_2 = ... = f_T = f_{LOE}$), and a distinct or smaller shifting factor value for the withdrawal due to adverse event ($f_1 = f_2 = ... = f_T = f_{AE}$). $f_{LOE} = f_{AE}$ is a special case. For loss to follow-up that is truly neutral to efficacy or safety, we may set the *shifting factor* ($f_1 = f_2 = ... = f_T = f_{NEU}$) equal to 0, which reduces to the MAR case. The effect of the NMAR data on the treatment comparison will naturally be dependent on the proportion of missing data in each pattern when performing the data analysis, which is the ω_j in Equation 10.13. These *shifting factors* (f_{LOE}, f_{AE}, f_{NEU}), which control the shift parameters Δ, are the *sensitivity parameters*. The parameters Δ and the baseline restriction for LOE (and/or AE) represent the presumption that a missing value due to LOE or AE would have a bad outcome if it were observed. This is especially true for, say, a pain score or blood pressure when the missing data is from a patient who discontinued the study treatment or took a rescue medication.

After all the MI steps under the NFD missingness are done, the usual statistical method for complete longitudinal data analysis can then be performed for each imputed set, and the results are integrated, for example, as performed by PROC MIANALYZE in SAS.

It is also a useful practice to display the sensitivity analysis by the summary of the efficacy results with different levels of the shifting factors. Table 10.3 illustrates a hypothetical example, using the p-values as the summary of efficacy results for different values of the sensitivity parameters (f_{LOE}, f_{AE}) with $f_{NEU} = 0$ and $f_{NEU} = 0.5$. If the conclusions are consistent within a reasonable range of the shifting parameters, then one can comfortably accept the result under the assumed model. Otherwise, the result will be subject to more scrutiny by skeptical reviewers.

Some practitioners also use ACT analysis as another kind of sensitivity analysis. However, strictly speaking, ACT analysis should not be regarded as a sensitivity analysis; rather, it should be regarded as a secondary analysis because it addresses a different estimand than the AAT estimand (Morris, Kahan, and White 2014). ACT analysis assumes that the dropouts from the treatment group would behave like those in the control (e.g., placebo) group, and the control has no effect, hence dropouts are all MAR, while AAT does

TABLE 10.3

Summary of Sensitivity Analyses: A Hypothetical Example
Using p-values as the Summary of Efficacy Results for
Different Values of the Sensitivity Parameters (f_{LOE}, f_{AE}, f_{NEU})

p-value	f_{LOE}				
$f_{NEU} = 0$					
f_{AE}	*0*	*0.5*	*0.75*	*1.0*	*1.2*
0	0.005	0.007	0.012	0.024	0.035
0.5	0.006	0.008	0.014	0.030	0.037
0.75	0.009	0.012	0.023	0.033	0.041
1.0	0.013	0.022	0.030	0.042	0.049
1.2	0.023	0.027	0.033	0.044	0.053
$f_{NEU} = 0.5$					
f_{AE}	*0.5*	*0.75*	*1.0*	*1.2*	
0.5	0.010	0.016	0.032	0.039	
0.75	0.014	0.025	0.035	0.043	
1.0	0.024	0.032	0.044	0.051	
1.2	0.029	0.035	0.046	0.055	

not make this assumption. The discrepancy in the results, if it appears, would then be attributed to the interpretation of the different estimands. ACT analysis is gaining popularity with the regulatory agencies because it is conservative, that is, it tends to shrink toward no treatment difference.

10.9 Other NMAR Approaches

An extensive literature also exists on other NMAR models. For example, a large class of NMAR is a special kind of random effects model where the missing data is assumed to depend on the underlying (unobserved) random effect, or latent variables. Sometimes, this class of NMAR is called shared parameter or random-coefficient-dependent models; see Molenberghs and Kenward (2007). Shih, Quan, and Chang (1994) illustrated the univariate case based on the simple random effect model introduced above in Section 4.5. They assumed that the MDM depends on the unobserved true value of the endpoint, instead of the potentially observed endpoint itself (Homework 10.5). In a sequence of papers, Wu and Bailey (1988, 1989), Wu and Carroll (1988), Schluchter (1992), Mori, Woodworth, and Woolson (1992), and Wu, Hunsberger, and Zucker (1994) developed methods of analyzing longitudinal data by using the rate of change (slope) as the estimand. The missing data due to dropouts is assumed to depend on the true (unobserved) underlying slope of the individual. For example, individuals with a gradual decrease of blood pressure tend to remain in the study, while those with an increase would drop out of the study prematurely. In this context, the term "informative right censoring" or "informative missing" data was used to mean that the MDM is not ignorable. The hazard of dropout in a shared parameter model will generally imply or directly result in a dependence of the missing data on future observations, even after conditioning on past and current observations. These models can be very useful for complex data structures, but because many layers of assumptions are needed for the model to fit the data, they have not been widely used in a regulatory setting. The sensitivity analysis in this class of NMAR models is an active and open research area.

Appendix 10.1: Sampling Distribution Inference

The inference is based on some (sufficient) statistic, say $S(V)$. To "ignore" the missing data usually means to fix $M = m$, the observed missing data pattern, and to compare the observed value of $S(V)$ to the distribution of $S(V)$ found from $S(V) = S(Y_o, m) = S(Y_o)$, that is, from the marginal distribution of Y_o alone: $[Y_o] = \int [Y]dY_m$. However, the correct reference distribution should be the conditional distribution of Y_o given M:

$$[Y_o \mid M] = \frac{\int [Y, M]dY_m}{[M]} = \frac{\int [M \mid Y][Y]dY_m}{\int [M \mid Y][Y]dY} \qquad (10A.1)$$

When $[M \mid Y]$ does not depend on Y, then we simplify the right-hand side of Equation 10A.1 and find $[Y_o \mid M] = \int [Y]dY_m, = [Y_o]$; in other words, "ignoring" the missing data is appropriate. The above condition "$[M \mid Y]$ does not depend on Y" is termed MCAR in the literature.

From the above discussion, we can see that a more precise way of saying "ignoring the missing data" should really be "ignoring the process that causes the missing data," because it is the $[M \mid Y]$ that is being ignored in Equation 10A.1.

In a clinical trial, if the cause of the missing data is not related to the observed or potential outcome of the patients, then MCAR may be assumed. Examples include patients who have moved away, the study ending, and late entry of patients being administratively "censored."

Appendix 10.2: Likelihood Inference

The inference is based on the likelihood function $L(\theta; V)$. When "ignoring" the missing data, we usually mean that $L(\theta; V) \propto [Y_o]$ for $\theta \in \Omega_\theta$ (the parameter space of θ), that is,

$$L(\theta; V) \propto \delta(\theta \in \Omega_\theta) \int [Y] dY_m \qquad (10A.2)$$

where δ is the indicator function.

However, the correct likelihood should be based on the joint distribution, that is, $L(\theta; V) \propto [Y_o, M]$ for $(\theta, \varphi) \in \Omega_\theta$ (the joint parameter space of θ and φ). Thus,

$$L(\theta; V) \propto \delta((\theta; \varphi) \in \Omega_{\theta,\varphi}) \int [M \,|\, Y][Y] dY_m \qquad (10A.3)$$

If (a) $\Omega_{\theta,\varphi} = \Omega_\theta \times \Omega_\varphi$ and (b) $[M|Y] = [M|Y_o]$, then Equation 10A.3 reduces to Equation 10A.2, and ignoring the missing data process is appropriate. The above condition (a) is termed *distinct parameters* (DP) and condition (b) is termed *missing at random* (MAR) in the literature. See discussion in Shih (1992).

In a longitudinal clinical trial, MAR may be assumed if the patient withdrawal from the study is due to the observed outcome in the past, not the current unobserved or future potential outcomes.

Appendix 10.3: Bayesian Inference

The discussion is similar to that in Appendix 10.2 with an extra prior distribution on the parameter space, $\Omega_{\theta,\varphi}$. The conditions for an ignorable missing data process are the same (a) and (b) as in Appendix 10.2.

The above "ignorability" discussion is naturally applicable to each treatment group, if we consider the conditional distribution $[Y|X_1]$ throughout the discussion, where X_1 denotes the treatment group, it can also be extended to conditioning on all predefined baseline covariates X. Second, the "ignorability" conditions given in the previous section are *sufficient conditions*. There may be other conditions by which the missing data process could also be ignorable. This is especially true when considering *testing* between treatment groups as opposed to the estimation within each treatment group parameters. The example in Section 10.4 illustrated a case where, under the null hypothesis that $\theta = 0$ (no treatment effect), the inference based on the observed data is unbiased. A discussion of sufficient conditions for *stratified testing* can be found in Shih and Quan (1998).

Appendix 10.4: Equivalence between Selection Model and Pattern-Mixture Model for MCAR and MAR

1. Rubin's (1976) definition of MCAR is based on the selection model factorization of the joint distribution of Y and M:

$$[Y, M] = [M|Y][Y] = [M][Y] \tag{10A.4}$$

when [M] does not depend on Y.

The pattern-mixture model, on the other hand, is based on a different factorization of the joint distribution of Y and M:

$$[Y, M] = [Y|M][M] \tag{10A.5}$$

For Equation 10A.4 = 10A.5, it follows that

$$[Y] = [Y|M] \tag{10A.6}$$

This is the MCAR under the pattern-mixture model, that is, the marginal distribution of Y is the same regardless of the pattern M. The reverse direction from Equation 10A.6 to implying [M|Y] = [M] is straightforward to show.

2. Rubin's (1976) definition of MAR is based on the selection model factorization of the joint distribution of Y and M:

$$[Y, M] = [M|Y][Y] = [M|Y_o, Y_m][Y] = [M|Y_o][Y] \tag{10A.7}$$

when $[M|Y_o, Y_m] = [M|Y_o]$, which is the selection model's condition of MAR.

Under this condition, Equation 10A.7 is written as

$$[Y_o, Y_m, M] = [M|Y_o][Y_o, Y_m]$$

$$= \frac{[Y_o|M][M]}{[Y_o]}[Y_o, Y_m]$$

$$= [Y_o|M][M]\frac{[Y_o, Y_m]}{[Y_o]} \tag{10A.8}$$

$$= [Y_o, M][Y_m|Y_o]$$

However, $[Y_o, Y_m, M] = [Y_o, M][Y_m|Y_o, M]$. Equating this to Equation 10A.8, we obtain

$$[Y_m|Y_o, M] = [Y_m|Y_o] \tag{10A.9}$$

Equation 10A.9 is the conditional of MAR with the pattern-mixture model approach. It says that the conditional distribution of Y_m given Y_o is independent of the pattern.

Conversely, starting from the pattern-mixture model approach, we factor

$$[Y, M] = [Y_o, Y_m, M] = [Y_o, M] [Y_m | Y_o, M]$$

Under the condition of Equation 10A.9,

$$[Y, M] = [Y_o, M] [Y_m | Y_o]$$

$$= [Y_o | M][M] \frac{[Y_m, Y_o]}{[Y_o]}$$

$$= \frac{[Y_o | M][M]}{[Y_o]} [Y_o, Y_m]$$

$$= [M | Y_o] [Y_o, Y_m]$$

$$= [M | Y_o] [Y]$$

We arrive at Equation 10A.7.

The equivalence of $[M | Y_o, Y_m] = [M | Y_o]$ (MAR under the selection model approach) and $[Y_m | Y_o, M] = [Y_m | Y_o]$ (MAR under the pattern-mixture model approach) has far-reaching implications. The selection model approach is useful for simulation studies to generate missing data with known mechanisms. The pattern-mixture model approach is useful for data analysis, where we can use the observed data to fit a predictive model of Y_m given Y_o (and other covariates and/or prior distribution of the parameters), from which the Y_m can then be sampled. This is the foundation of the MI method.

Appendix 10.5: NFD Missingness Mechanism as a Subclass of NMAR for Longitudinal Data with Monotone Missing Data Pattern

With the selection model setting, we factor $[Y, M] = [M | Y][Y] = [M | Yo, Ym][Y]$. When the MDM $[M | Y] = [M | Y_o, Y_m]$ depends not only on Y_o (as for MAR) but also on the missing data Y_m, it is called NMAR or MNAR. As there are infinitely many different ways M can depend on Y_m, we shall further subclass the NMAR models. For longitudinal data with Y_k, $k = 0, 1, 2, \ldots T$, where $k = 0$ is the baseline visit, following the monotone missing data pattern characterized by $L = 0, 1, \ldots, T$, as described in Section 10.6, the above selection model factorization is then written as

$$[Y_0, Y_1, \ldots, Y_j, \ldots, Y_T, L = j] = [L = j | Y_0, Y_1, \ldots, Y_j, \ldots, Y_T] [Y_0, Y_1, \ldots, Y_j, \ldots, Y_T]$$

Recall that L is the last visit during which a subject has a measurement observed. If the MDM is such that

$$[L = j | Y_0, Y_1, \ldots, Y_j, \ldots, Y_T] = [L = j | Y_0, Y_1, \ldots, Y_{j+1}] \qquad (10A.10)$$

it is then called NFD missingness; in other words, the current unobserved outcome Y_{j+1} (for the pattern $L = j$) depends on the past observed outcomes $(Y_1, \ldots, Y_j)$ as well as the presently missing outcome Y_{j+1} (itself), but not on the future outcomes $(Y_{j+2}, \ldots, Y_T)$. (Kenward, Molenberghs, and Thijs 2003).

This NFD missingness is a subclass of the NMAR. NFD missingness includes MAR as a special case, because it adds one more restriction on the missing mechanism in addition to that for MAR.

This definition of NFD missingness, expressed by the MDM (Equation 10A.10) is with the selection model framework and is very intuitive. However, for analyzing data, it is more convenient to use the pattern-mixture model approach (see Equation 10A.13). With the pattern-mixture framework, NFD missingness has another form, defined by Kenward, Molenberghs, and Thijs (2003) as follows:

Assume that the baseline value Y_0 is always observed, and that the first missing data occurs at the first follow-up visit. (If the first missing data occurs at a visit beyond the first follow-up visit, then we can let Y_0 be a vector of observed visits, for easier notation.) The NFD missingness is such that, for all follow-up visits $k \geq 2$ and all patterns $j < k-1$

$$[Y_k | Y_0, Y_1 \ldots, Y_{k-1}, L = j] = [Y_k | Y_0, Y_1, \ldots, Y_{k-1}, L \geq k-1] \qquad (10A.11)$$

It can be shown that the condition in Equation 10A.11 is equivalent to

$$[Y_k | Y_0, Y_1 \ldots, Y_{k-1}, L = j] = [Y_k | Y_0, Y_1, \ldots, Y_{k-1}] \qquad (10A.12)$$

The proof uses similar steps as in Appendix 10.4b and is assigned as a homework problem (Homework 10.3).

Another homework assignment is to show the equivalence between Equations 10A.10 and 10A.12; see Appendix 10.6.

Note that with the NFD missing data condition (Equation 10A.11), the distribution $[Y_k | Y_0, Y_1, \ldots, Y_{k-1}, L = k-1]$ was left unspecified for $k = 1, \ldots, T$.

We need to make an assumption for this unidentified model to proceed. As in the MAR case, we link it with the $L > k$ patterns where Y_{k+1}
is observed. One such an assumption is the mean shift model as a simple
departure from MAR, as discussed in Section 10.7. This assumption is not
verifiable from the observed data and requires sensitivity analyses for
varying shift values.

Specifically, we write the whole joint distribution with the pattern-mixture
factorization

$$[Y_0, Y_1, ..., Y_j, ..., Y_T, L = j] = [Y_0, Y_1, ..., Y_j, ..., Y_T | L = j] [L = j] \qquad (10A.13)$$

The pattern-specific joint distribution $[Y_0, Y_1, ..., Y_j, ..., Y_T | L = j]$ can be
written as

$$[Y_0, Y_1, ..., Y_j, ..., Y_T | L = j] = [Y_0, Y_1, ..., Y_j | L = j] [Y_{j+1} | Y_0, Y_1, ..., Y_j, L = j]$$

$$\times \prod_{k=j+2}^{T} [Y_k | Y_0, Y_1, ..., Y_{k-1}, L = j] \qquad (10A.14)$$

The first factor of Equation 10A.14 is clearly identifiable from the observed
data. The second and beyond are not identified due to the missing data
and require additional assumptions. The second factor could be identified
by linking it to the observed $[Y_{j+1} | Y_0, Y_1, ..., Y_j, L \geq j+1]$ with an additional
assumption. (The special shift parameter model is a simple yet useful way
to link.) The third and beyond factors could be identified with the help of
the NFD condition (Equation 10A.11) together with the same link as for the
second factor as follows: Using Equation 10A.11, for $k \geq j+2$,

$$[Y_k | Y_0, Y_1, ..., Y_{k-1}, L = j] = [Y_k | Y_0, Y_1, ..., Y_{k-1}, L \geq k-1]$$

Furthermore, the right-hand side $[Y_k | Y_0, Y_1, ..., Y_{k-1}, L \geq k-1]$

$$= \sum_{s=k-1}^{T} \frac{[Y_0, Y_1, ..., Y_{k-1}, L = s]}{[Y_0, Y_1, ..., Y_{k-1}, L \geq k-1]} [Y_k | Y_0, Y_1, ..., Y_{k-1}, L = s] \qquad (10A.15)$$

and $\quad \dfrac{[Y_0, Y_1, ..., Y_{k-1}, L = s]}{[Y_0, Y_1, ..., Y_{k-1}, L \geq k-1]} = \dfrac{P(L = s)[Y_0, Y_1, ..., Y_{k-1} | L = s]}{\sum_{s=k-1}^{T} P(L = s)[Y_0, Y_1, ..., Y_{k-1} | L = s]}$

Note that $[Y_0, Y_1, ..., Y_{k-1} | L = s]$ can be identified from the observed data
for $s \geq k-1$. $[Y_k | Y_0, Y_1, ..., Y_{k-1}, L = s]$ can be identified from the observed
data for $s \geq k$. The unidentified $[Y_k | Y_0, Y_1, ..., Y_{k-1}, L = k-1]$ is linked

to $[Y_k | Y_0, Y_1, ..., Y_{k-1}, L \geq k]$ by the same shift model as for the second factor. Thus, all factors in Equation 10A.14 can be identified. The mean shift model as a simple yet useful way to describe the departure from MAR is expressed as

$$E[Y_k | Y_0, Y_1, ..., Y_{k-1}, L = k-1] = E[Y_k | Y_0, Y_1, ..., Y_{k-1}, L \geq k] + \Delta_k$$

An example for $T = 4$ is given in Section 10.7 for illustration.

Appendix 10.6: Equivalence between the Selection Model NFD Missingness Condition (Equation 10A.10) and the Pattern-Mixture Model NFD Missingness Condition (Equation 10A.12)

The proof is given in the study by Peng (2015) (Homework 10.4).

Homework 10.1

Generate a longitudinal data set with MAR missing values by the selection model specification and analyze the trend.

1. Consider the following model. First, the complete data is a sequence $\{Y_t : t = 1, ..., 10\}$ from a multivariate normal distribution with $E(Y_t) = \alpha_0 + \alpha_1 t$ and covariance matrix $(1 - \rho)I + \rho J$, that is, variances $= 1$ at each t and the correlation between Y_s and Y_t equals ρ for all $t \neq s$. (See the parameters values below.) Second, the monotone missing pattern and the MDM are defined as follows. Let L be the last time point t at which Y_t is observed. Let $\Pr(L = j+1 | Y_1, ..., Y_j, L \geq j+1) = p(Y_j | L \geq j+1)$, and set $\log[p(y)/(1 - p(y))] = \beta_0 + \beta_1 y$. That is, we assume a logistic regression model for the monotone MDM that the chance of missing or observing at $t = j+1$ depends only on the last observed value at $t = j$. Finally, generate a set of $n = 100$ realizations of the above process by assuming the correlation $\rho = 0.9$, $\alpha_0 = 1$, $\alpha_1 = 0$ (i.e., no trend), $\beta_0 = -1$, and $\beta_1 = -2$. Note that, using the notation of the selection model factorization (Equation 10.1), $\theta = (\alpha_0, \alpha_1, \rho)$ and $\varphi = (\beta_0, \beta_1)$. This model satisfies both MAR and DP (distinct parameters) conditions. Plot the generated data. As a sampling-distribution-based inference (see Appendix 10.1), connect the sample mean values at each time point $t = 1, ..., 10$. Comment on and explain what you see about the empirical trend.

2. As a likelihood-based inference (see Appendix 10.2), use PROC MIXED and use PROC MI and PROC ANALYZE to analyze the above generated data and estimate the true trend α_1. Comment on your estimates (one from single imputation PROC MIXED and another from multiple imputation PROC MI) in contrast to the empirical trend in (a).

3. Do the same as above but change to $\rho = 0$. Again, compare the estimated trend with the empirical trend.

Homework 10.2

Generate a longitudinal data set with NMAR-NFD missing values and analyze the data.

1. The complete data model and the monotone pattern are the same as above, but use the following MDM model: $Pr(L = j+1|Y_1, ..., Y_j, L \geq j+1) = p(Y_{j+1}|L \geq j+1)$, and $\log[p(y)/(1-p(y))] = \beta_0 + \beta_1 y$. That is, the chance of missing or observing at $t = j + 1$ depends on only the current value at $t = j+1$. Use the same parameter values for $\rho = 0.9$, $\alpha_0 = 1$, $\alpha_1 = 0$, $\beta_0 = -1$, and $\beta_1 = -2$. Plot the realization set of data for $n = 100$.

2. Conduct the pattern-mixture model approach with Δ_k shift set to be within one RSD of Y_t given $Y_1, ..., Y_{t-1}$ (estimated from the imputed complete data under MAR), as described in Section 10.7. Use the single adjustment, nonrecursive/nonsequential and recursive/sequential procedures to estimate the marginal means $E(Y_t)$ at each time point $t = 1$ to 10 and compare their results.

Homework 10.3

Derive Equation 10A.12 from Equation 10A.11. (Hint: Use similar steps as in Appendix 10.4b.)

Homework 10.4

Prove the assertion in Appendix 10.6. (Hint: Use induction.)

Homework 10.5

Consider a two-stage random effect model for $Y = \{y_i, i = 1, ..., N\}$

$$y_i | \mu_i \sim N(\mu_i, \sigma^2)$$

$$\mu_i | \mu \sim N(\mu, \tau^2)$$

where y_i is the response (e.g., change from baseline), μ_i is the true (unobserved) response of the ith subject, σ^2 is the within-subject variance and τ^2 is the between-subject variance. Note that this is related to the model (Equation 4.20) in Section 4.5. Our interest is to estimate μ, the group mean response. Suppose $Y_o = \{y_1, ..., y_n\}$ are observed, and the rest $Y_m = \{y_{n+1}, ..., y_N\}$ are missing. Use a question mark to denote missing values. We assume the MDM to follow $\Pr(y_i = ? | \mu_i) = I(\mu_i < c)$ for some constant c, where I(.) is the indicator function. That is, when the true change is less than c, then the response is not observed. Note that μ_i is always unobservable.

1. Corresponding to Y, let $M = \{m_i, i = 1, ..., N\}$ be the missing data pattern for Y; $m_i = 1$ when y_i is observed and 0 otherwise. The MDM can be written as $g(m_i | y_i, \mu_i) = I\{I(\mu_i > c) - m_i = 0\}$. Argue that this MDM is a nonignorable case.

2. If one ignores the (nonignorable) MDM, and uses the sample mean $\bar{Y}_n$ to estimate μ, show that when N increases, but n/N remains constant, the asymptotic bias of $\bar{Y}_n$ is

$$\bar{Y}_n - \mu = \frac{N\tau}{n\sqrt{2\pi}} \exp\left\{-\frac{1}{2}\left[\Phi^{-1}\left(\frac{N-n}{N}\right)\right]^2\right\} > 0$$

where Φ^{-1} is the inverse of the cdf of the standard normal distribution.

References

CDER (US Department of Health and Human Services, Food and Drug Administration, Center for Drug Evaluation and Research). (2014). *Guidance for Industry—Analgesic Indications: Developing Drug and Biological Products (Draft Guidance)*. http://www.fda.gov/Drugs/GuidanceComplianceRegulatoryInformation/Guidances/default.htm (accessed on March 31, 2014).

Choi SC and Lu IL. (1995). Effect of non-random missing data mechanisms in clinical trials. *Statistics in Medicine* 14: 2675–2684. doi:10.1002/sim.4780142407.

Daniels MJ and Hogan JW. (2007). *Missing Data in Longitudinal Studies: Strategies for Bayesian Modeling and Sensitivity Analysis*. Boca Raton, FL: Chapman & Hall/ CRC Press.

Diggle PJ and Shih WJ. (1993). On informative and random dropouts in longitudinal studies. *Biometrics* 49: 947–949.

EMEA (European Medicines Evaluation Agency). (1998). *Statistical Principles for Clinical Trials; Step 5: Note for Guidance on Statistical Principles for Clinical Trials*. International Conference on Harmonisation (ICH) Topic E9. http://www.ema. europa.eu/docs/en_GB/document_library/Scientific_guideline/2009/09/ WC500002928.pdf (accessed on April 21, 2015).

Finkelstein D and Schoenfeld D. (1999). Combining mortality and longitudinal measures in clinical trials. *Statistics in Medicine* 18: 1341–1354.

Kenward MG, Molenberghs G, and Thijs H. (2003). Pattern-mixture models with proper time dependence. *Biometrika* 90: 53–71.

Laird NM and Ware JH. (1982). Random-effects models for longitudinal data. *Biometrics* 38: 963–74.

Liang KY and Zeger SL. (1986). Longitudinal data analysis using generalized linear models. *Biometrika* 73: 13–22.

Little RJA. (1993). Pattern-mixture models for multivariate incomplete data. *Journal of the American Statistical Association* 88: 125–134.

Little RJA. (1995). Modeling the drop-out mechanism in repeated-measures studies. *Journal of the American Statistical Association* 90: 1112–1121.

Little RJA and Yao L. (1998). Statistical techniques for analyzing data from prevention trials: treatment of no-shows using Rubin's causal model. *Psychological Methods* 3: 147–159.

Little RJA, Cohen ML, Dickersin K, Emerson SS, Farrar JT, Neaton JD, Shih WJ, et al. (2012a). The design and conduct of clinical trials to limit missing data. *Statistics in Medicine*. July 2012. doi:10.1002/sim.5519.

Little RJA, Cohen ML, Dickersin K, Emerson SS, Farrar JT, Neaton JD, Shih, WJ, et al. (2012b). The prevention and treatment of missing data in clinical trials. *New England Journal of Medicine* 367: 1355–1360. October 4, 2012. doi:10.1056/NEJM sr1203730.

Molenberghs G and Kenward MG. (2007). *Missing Data in Clinical Studies*. Chichester, UK: Wiley.

Mori M, Woodworth G, and Woolson RF. (1992). Application of empirical bayes methodology to estimation of changes in the presence of informative right censoring. *Statistics in Medicine* 11: 621–631.

Morris TP, Kahan BC, and White IR. (2014). Choosing sensitivity analyses for randomised trials: principles. *BMC Medical Research Methodology* 14: 11 doi:10.1186/1471-2288-14-11.

NRC (National Research Council). (2010). *The Prevention and Treatment of Missing Data in Clinical Trials*. Panel on Handling Missing Data in Clinical Trials. Committee on National Statistics, Division of Behavioral and Social Sciences and Education. Washington, DC: The National Academies Press.

Paik MC. (1997). The generalized estimating equation approach when data are not missing completely at random. *Journal of the American Statistical Association* 92: 1320–1329.

Peng L. (2015). Design of Primary and Sensitivity Analysis of Non-Future Dependence Missing Data in Clinical Trials With an Emphasis on the Type-I

Error Rate Using Multiple Imputation and Pattern Mixture Model Approach. Ph.D. Dissertation, Department of Biostatistics, Rutgers School of Public Health, Rutgers University, The State University of New Jersey.

Ratitch B, O'Kelly M, and Tosielloc R. (2013). Missing data in clinical trials: from clinical assumptions to statistical analysis using pattern mixture models. *Pharmaceutical Statistics* (wileyonlinelibrary.com) doi:10.1002/pst.1549.

Robins JM, Rotnitzky A, and Zhao LP. (1995). Analysis of semiparametric regression models for repeated outcomes in the presence of missing data. *Journal of the American Statistical Association* 90: 106–121.

Rubin DB. (1976). Inference and missing data. *Biometrika* 63: 581–592.

Rubin DB. (1998). Multiple imputation for nonresponse in surveys. New York: Wiley.

SAS® Institute. SAS/STAT® procedure release 9.2, PROC MIXED, PROC MI, PROC MIANALYZE.

Schafer JL. (1997). *Analysis of Incomplete Multivariate Data.* New York: Chapman and Hall.

Schluchter MD. (1992). Methods for the analysis of informatively censoring longitudinal data. *Statistics in Medicine* 11: 1861–1870.

Shih WJ. (1992). On informative and random dropouts in longitudinal studies. *Biometrics* 48: 970–972.

Shih WJ, Quan H, and Chang MN. (1994). Estimation of the mean when data contain non-ignorable missing values from a random effects model. *Statistics & Probability Letters* 19: 249–257.

Shih WJ and Quan H. (1998). Stratified testing for treatment effects with missing data. *Biometrics* 54: 782–787.

Yuan YC. (2001). Multiple Imputation for Missing Data: Concepts and New Development SAS/STAT® 8.2. [http://www.sas.com/statistics]. Cary, NC: SAS Institute.

Wu MC and Bailey KR. (1988). Analyzing changes in the presence of informative right censoring caused by death and withdrawal. *Statistics in Medicine* 7: 337–346.

Wu MC and Carroll RJ. (1988). Estimation and comparison of changes in the presence of informative right censoring by codeling the censoring process. *Biometrics* 44: 175–188.

Wu MC and Bailey KR. (1989). Estimation and comparison of changes in the presence of informative right censoring: conditional linear model. *Biometrics* 45: 939–955.

Wu MC, Hunsberger S, and Zucker D. (1994). Testing differences in changes in the presence of censoring: parametric and nonparametric methods. *Statistics in Medicine* 13: 635–646.

Index

Printed in the United States
by Baker & Taylor Publisher Services